"Robert Davis cuts through the fat and clears up the confusion about the diet and nutrition issues on everyone's minds in this unique, concise, easy-to-read book. *Coffee Is Good for You* will educate you, entertain you, and even make you laugh. A must-read for anyone who's ever wondered whether or not to believe the hype."

—Lisa "Hungry Girl" Lillien

"Robert Davis deftly blends wit, wisdom, keen insights, and a voice of unfailing reason. I will be recommending this great resource to everyone I know."

—Dr. David Katz,
director of the Yale University Prevention Research Center

"Wow, that was easy to understand! Robert Davis does it again with his lighthearted and sensible translation of complicated nutrition science into simple how-to messages on healthy eating. Who knew reading about nutrition research could be so much fun?"

—Carolyn O'Neil, MS, RD, coauthor of *The Dish*

"This book is a gem. With clarity, wit, and wisdom, Robert Davis debunks medical myths and gives the reader real information to rely on. This book is stuffed with nuggets and is a great read. It's as well referenced as most medical school textbooks . . . just a lot more fun."

—Dr. Nancy Snyderman, NBC News Chief Medical Editor

Coffee Is B~~ad~~ *good* for You

From Vitamin C and Organic Foods to Low-Carb and Detox Diets, the Truth About Diet and Nutrition Claims

Robert J. Davis, PhD

A PERIGEE BOOK

A PERIGEE BOOK
Published by the Penguin Group
Penguin Group (USA) Inc.
375 Hudson Street, New York, New York 10014, USA

Penguin Group (Canada), 90 Eglinton Avenue East, Suite 700, Toronto, Ontario M4P 2Y3, Canada (a division of Pearson Penguin Canada Inc.) • Penguin Books Ltd., 80 Strand, London WC2R 0RL, England • Penguin Group Ireland, 25 St. Stephen's Green, Dublin 2, Ireland (a division of Penguin Books Ltd.) • Penguin Group (Australia), 250 Camberwell Road, Camberwell, Victoria 3124, Australia (a division of Pearson Australia Group Pty. Ltd.) • Penguin Books India Pvt. Ltd., 11 Community Centre, Panchsheel Park, New Delhi—110 017, India • Penguin Group (NZ), 67 Apollo Drive, Rosedale, Auckland 0632, New Zealand (a division of Pearson New Zealand Ltd.) • Penguin Books (South Africa) (Pty.) Ltd., 24 Sturdee Avenue, Rosebank, Johannesburg 2196, South Africa

Penguin Books Ltd., Registered Offices: 80 Strand, London WC2R 0RL, England

While the author has made every effort to provide accurate telephone numbers and Internet addresses at the time of publication, neither the publisher nor the author assumes any responsibility for errors or for changes that occur after publication. Further, the publisher does not have any control over and does not assume any responsibility for author or third-party websites or their content.

Copyright © 2012 by Robert J. Davis, PhD, MPH
The *New Yorker* caption on page 144 is used with permission. Copyright © by Alex Gregory/The New Yorker Collection/www.cartoonbank.com.
Text design by Ellen Cipriano

Library of Congress Cataloging-in-Publication Data

ISBN 978-0-399-53725-7

PRINTED IN THE UNITED STATES OF AMERICA

PUBLISHER'S NOTE: Neither the publisher nor the author is engaged in rendering professional advice or services to the individual reader. The ideas, procedures, and suggestions contained in this book are not intended as a substitute for consulting with your physician. All matters regarding your health require medical supervision. Neither the author nor the publisher shall be liable or responsible for any loss or damage allegedly arising from any information or suggestion in this book.

For Emily

Contents

Introduction

Though food is supposed to be one of life's simple pleasures, few things cause more angst and confusion. It's no wonder why. We're constantly being told which foods we should eat to be healthy, which diets we should follow to be skinny, which preparation methods we should use to be safe, and which chemicals and contaminants in food we should shun to avoid illness. It's enough to give anyone indigestion.

This hullabaloo over food is nothing new. In 1910, the *Washington Post* published an article railing against popular diet and nutrition advice. "Of all subjects," said the article, "that of food is the most apt to be the riding ground of cranks."

To set the record straight, the article proceeded to provide one physician's list of 39 "false food fads." These so-called myths included:

- Candy and sugar are bad for you.
- Vegetables with stalks and leaves are nutritious.
- Meals should last more than 30 minutes.
- The average American eats too much.

On the contrary, this expert said, sugar is "one of the cheapest and best forms of nourishment," vegetables such as celery and broccoli lack nutrients, "dawdling over meals" is bad for you, and many people don't eat enough. Hmm. I guess by his reasoning, the millions of us today who constantly stuff ourselves with quick, sugar-laden meals, while never touching broccoli or spinach, have the right idea.

Maybe the paper would have done its readers a greater service by publishing the views of the "cranks."

Separating the cranks from the credible sources is even tougher today than it was 100 years ago. In a recent survey by the U.S. Food and Drug Administration (FDA), more than two thirds of Americans agreed with the statement that "there are so many recommendations about healthy ways to eat, it is hard for me to know what to believe." We face a barrage of dietary information from the news media, food companies, health groups, government agencies, celebrities, diet-book authors, and of course the Internet, which gives every self-proclaimed expert the ability to reach a worldwide audience with just a few keystrokes.

Often this advice is maddeningly contradictory. Coffee is bad for you. No, wait, it's good. Fiber prevents colon cancer. No, it doesn't. Fat is what causes weight gain. No, it's carbs. Eat according to the government's food pyramid. Never mind, make that a plate. The list goes on and on.

If you're confused about what to believe, you've come to the right place. In *Coffee Is Good for You*, I'll give you the bottom line on an array of popular diet and nutrition claims in a quick, easily digestible way.

As a health journalist, I'm called on to do this all the time. Whether at home or work, at speeches I give or social gatherings I attend, I find myself constantly answering questions about diet and health. Dinners with friends and relatives seem incomplete unless someone at some point shoves a box, bottle, or carton in my face and asks whether whatever it contains is okay to consume.

Ironically, our growing confusion comes at a time when scientists who study nutrition know more than ever. The field has advanced rapidly in the past few decades, providing an unprecedented level of knowledge about what's good and bad for us.

So why the disconnect? For starters, we usually learn about diet and health in bits and pieces that can be misleading. The media, our main source of information on the subject, typically report on scientific advances in short snippets devoid of context. It's like being shown a single piece of a jigsaw puzzle. We have no idea how big the piece is relative to the others, where it fits in, or, for that matter, what the picture is supposed to be.

Similarly, when we hear about a study in isolation, it's hard to draw accurate conclusions. Just because one piece of research shows, for example, that prunes make your ears floppy doesn't necessarily mean it's true. Yet if the media portray the study as definitive and fail to put the information in context, we can end up believing that prunes are bad for us.

Then when another study finds that prunes are safe, we feel confused and frustrated because scientists can't seem to make up their minds. But the problem doesn't lie with science or scientists. Rather, it lies with the misinterpretation of science—premature conclusions based on one piece of a puzzle.

Our confusion also stems from advice peddlers' selective use of science. Many who advise us about diet and nutrition have an agenda—whether selling a product, pushing a weight-loss regimen, or simply trying to get attention—and they misleadingly pick and choose studies to help further their cause. A company promoting its exotic fruit drink, for example, may claim that the ingredients have been tested and proven to help you shed pounds. Sounds convincing unless you know that the test subjects happened to be fat rats and the results may not apply to people.

In this book, I'll take you beyond the snippets and agendas, providing a thorough and unbiased look at what the science really says about food and health claims that we often hear. Think of me as a nutrition umpire—someone who can size up the claims and call balls and strikes without fear or favor. I do so relying on my academic training in epidemiology and biostatistics as well as my 20-plus years of experience reporting on nutrition and health.

I'll focus on claims that come up especially often in questions I'm asked and nutrition advice I encounter. While you won't find answers here to every question you have about diet and health, I hope that many of them will be addressed. And I suspect you'll often find the answers surprising.

CLIMBING THE PYRAMID

Before I explain my method for evaluating claims, a word on how nutrition studies are conducted. While this may seem a bit dry and technical, bear with me. The information is crucial for making

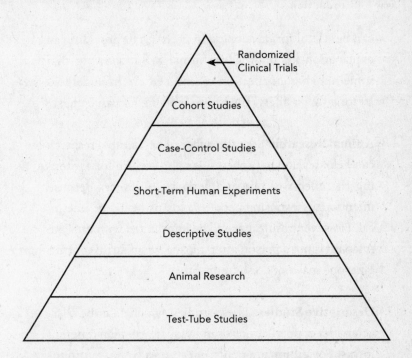

Randomized Clinical Trials

Cohort Studies

Case-Control Studies

Short-Term Human Experiments

Descriptive Studies

Animal Research

Test-Tube Studies

sense of the science. A basic understanding of scientific studies will not only help you understand how I arrived at my conclusions but also arm you to make your own informed judgments about food and nutrition claims.

Not all studies are created equal. Some are more credible than others. In fact, there's a hierarchy of evidence, which is sometimes shown as a pyramid. The higher you go, the greater the potential for definitive answers.

Let's start at the bottom and work our way up.

Test-Tube Studies: Also known as in vitro studies, these involve cells and tissues from humans or animals. They can be useful for developing hypotheses or providing an explanation for findings in humans. But showing that something has an effect on cells is a far cry from demonstrating that it affects the health of living human beings.

Animal Research: Like test-tube studies, animal research can help develop hypotheses. It's also well suited for testing the effects of potentially toxic substances because intentionally exposing people to toxins would be unethical. However, results have to be interpreted with caution. A lab rat is not a person after all, and what harms (or benefits) one may not do so to the other.

Descriptive Studies: These studies, which describe characteristics of populations or individuals, come in different forms. For example, population studies compare groups from various geographic locations, looking for differences in disease rates and in some dietary habit (such as fat intake) that might be responsible. Cross-sectional studies take a snapshot, reporting dietary habits and illness rates at a given time within a single population. Descriptive studies can show correlations, but they can't demonstrate cause and effect. It's possible that some other, unmeasured factor is actually responsible for any apparent connection.

Short-Term Human Experiments: In these trials, small numbers of human subjects are assigned to consume the food in question. After hours, days, or weeks, researchers measure some marker, such as the level of a particular substance in the blood, to see if any changes have occurred. In some cases, there's a comparison group that didn't eat the food. While such studies can provide hints about a food's effect on disease, they're considered preliminary. A short-term change in a marker doesn't necessarily translate into higher or lower rates of disease.

Case-Control Studies: These are a relatively quick and inexpensive way to test hypotheses generated by other types of studies down the pyramid. Researchers select two groups that are similar except that members of one (the cases) have a particular condition, and people in the other (the controls) don't. Information is then gathered about subjects' past eating habits to see if there are differences that might explain the disparity in disease. While case-control studies can reveal associations, they can't prove causation. One potential problem is that people may have fuzzy memories when asked to recall their eating habits. It's also possible that the two groups aren't as similar as the researchers believe and that some other factor, besides the food in question, really explains the illness among cases.

Cohort Studies: In contrast to case-control studies, cohort studies start with healthy people and are typically forward looking. People are asked about their dietary habits and then followed for years or decades to see who gets the condition(s) in question and who doesn't. Though they can't prove causality, findings from large, well-designed cohort studies can provide strong circumstantial evidence. Much of what we know about diet and health comes from large, long-term cohort studies, like the Nurses' Health Study led by researchers at Harvard.

Randomized Clinical Trials: These are the gold standard of studies, the only type capable of proving cause and effect. Subjects are randomly assigned to either follow a particular diet or not. If a dietary supplement is being tested, subjects get either the supplement or a placebo. The two groups are then followed for an extended period (often years) to see whether they fare differently. While randomized trials are useful for testing supplements, they're trickier when it comes to diet because people don't always eat exactly what's prescribed. Because of the complexity and expense involved, it often isn't feasible to test foods or dietary patterns with randomized trials. Plus, they're inappropriate if the food or supplement in question is suspected of causing harm, because asking people to consume it would be unethical.

A type of research not on the pyramid is a *systematic review*—a study of studies that examines an entire body of evidence on a subject to draw conclusions. In short, it looks at all the pieces of the puzzle and tries to put them together. Sometimes this process may involve a *meta-analysis*, a technique for pooling data from different studies. Although systematic reviews, like all research, can be biased or flawed, a well-conducted review can be a very powerful tool for assessing the overall strength and quality of the evidence.

THE TRUTH SCALE

Research about diet and health rarely yields the equivalent of DNA evidence, which provides incontrovertible proof. All types of studies—even randomized trials—come with caveats. However, if interpreted properly, a body of research can allow us to make sound judgments about how believable a claim is.

To that end, I've carefully reviewed the relevant studies (which are listed in the reference section in case you'd like to check them out for yourself) and assigned each claim to one of four categories on what I call the Truth Scale:

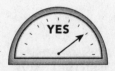

This means the claim is believable because there's solid supporting evidence from the top of the pyramid—at least several randomized trials or large cohort studies with consistent results. As a whole, other evidence points in the same direction.

This indicates the claim is half true. It contains an element of truth because some aspect of it is supported by solid science. For example, the claim may be valid for a limited number of people or in limited circumstances. But overall, it's misleading.

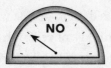

This means the claim is not believable based on the available evidence. The supporting research may be very limited or nonexistent. If there's a body of research, the bulk of it—especially from the top of the pyramid—refutes the claim, or indisputable scientific facts shoot it down.

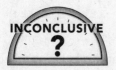

This signifies a scientific gray zone. Research overall is conflicting, or there's enough evidence from the middle of the pyramid to suggest that the claim could have merit but not enough to warrant a thumbs-up.

As you read through my takes on claims, here are a few things to keep in mind:

Funding sources matter. Increasingly, diet and nutrition studies are funded by food manufacturers, produce growers, weight-loss companies, and supplement makers. Corporate sponsorship doesn't necessarily mean the results are invalid, but it does at least raise the possibility that the study was somehow influenced to favor the funder's agenda. One analysis of studies on soft drinks, juices, and milk, for example, found that the studies funded by the food industry were more likely to report positive findings for the sponsor than those without industry funding. In assessing the research, I have relied whenever possible on studies supported by neutral entities such as the National Institutes of Health.

Effects are generally small. Studies often report findings as relative risks (RRs). An RR of 2.0 in a cohort study, for example, means that eating food X is associated with twice the risk of disease Y. Relative risks in nutrition studies are frequently less than 2, which is considered fairly small. (By comparison, the RR of lung cancer among male smokers is 23.) Small RRs don't mean that the potential harms (or benefits) from foods are inconsequential, just that they're generally limited. For the most part I have refrained from listing RRs because they provide no insight into what our actual risk is (two times higher than what?) and are easily misinterpreted.

Flip-flops aren't all bad. It can be frustrating when we repeatedly hear that something like coffee, eggs, or fat is bad for us, only to be told later, "never mind." In some cases, the inconsistencies stem from taking isolated studies out of context and misinterpreting research in the way I described earlier. But in others, the reversals occur because scientists have newer, better information. If you think about it, that's how science is supposed to work: It's constantly expanding what we know and inching us closer to the truth. As a result, some of what you read here will undoubtedly be superseded by new information in the future.

HEY, I'M JUST THE UMP

During a talk I gave several years ago, a young woman in the audience raised her hand to ask about a dietary supplement she was taking. As I explained that the evidence was limited and what we did know wasn't very promising, I could see her hopeful expression turn into a scowl. Clearly, it wasn't the answer she wanted to hear. When I finished, she responded curtly, "Well, I don't really trust studies."

Certainly, scientific research isn't perfect. And insufficient evidence doesn't necessarily mean a claim is false. It's possible that with more research, the supplement in which the woman placed so much faith might eventually be proven effective.

Still, modern scientific research is the best tool we have for separating facts from beliefs about diet and nutrition. If we reject it, we're left with faith, hunches, and anecdotes—the things that people like that expert in the newspaper were forced to rely on 100 years ago. And we saw what that got them.

My goal is to help you put scientific research to use so you can make informed decisions for yourself and your family. Like an umpire, I'll apply the rules and make the calls as accurately and honestly as I can. Unlike an umpire, though, I have no power of enforcement. It's up to you to decide whether and when to abide by my calls. Keep that in mind if, like my scowling questioner, you feel an urge to boo and throw food at the ump.

Chapter 1

Driven to Drink

COFFEE IS BAD FOR YOU

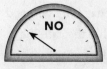 I'm not sure why I don't like coffee. Maybe it's the memory of my grandmother downing multiple cups of cheap instant coffee every morning as she sucked on one cigarette after another. It all seemed downright disgusting to me as a child, and I remember thinking that if this is what adults do, then maybe I shouldn't grow up.

When people learn that I don't drink coffee, they sometimes look at me as though I have an extra head. Over the years, I've learned how to allay their suspicions: I attribute my avoidance to health concerns about coffee. That way, my lack of conformity seems like a virtue.

Unfortunately, I can't get away with that excuse anymore. There's scant evidence that coffee is harmful. Indeed, it may even be good for us.

Coffee's unhealthy reputation stems in part from older studies linking java to an increased risk of heart disease and pancreatic cancer, among other things. But that research failed to account for smoking, which as my grandmother could have told the scientists was once coffee's constant companion.

More recent cohort studies, which followed tens of thousands of people for many years, have found that coffee drinkers have no greater risk of heart attacks or strokes; indeed, they appear to have a slightly lower risk. Ditto for type 2 diabetes and gout.

As for cancer, the research overall shows that coffee does not increase the risk, and it's even been associated with lower odds of certain cancers. What's more, coffee drinkers appear to live just as long as abstainers—and maybe even slightly longer.

One possible reason for these apparent benefits is that coffee is rich in antioxidants. But what about caffeine? That can't be good for you, can it? Indeed, some research suggests that the caffeine in coffee and other beverages may increase the risk of miscarriages, but the evidence overall is mixed. Generally, a cup or two a day (up to 200 milligrams of caffeine) appears to be safe during pregnancy.

Research has also linked more than three cups a day of caffeinated coffee to bone fractures among women who get too little calcium. And caffeine can cause jitters, insomnia, and stomach upset in some people. On the other hand, caffeinated coffee has been associated with a lower risk of Parkinson's disease.

For many people, the biggest health risk from coffee is weight gain. Though a cup of black coffee has only two calories, those Double Chocolaty Chip Frappuccinos and other blended beverages from coffee shops can quickly pack on extra pounds if you're not careful. Hey, maybe that's my new excuse for skipping the trips to Starbucks: I'm on a diet.

Decaf coffee typically contains some caffeine. Research shows that certain decaf beverages—such as lattes—can have as much caffeine as a can of soda.

RED WINE IS THE MOST BENEFICIAL TYPE OF ALCOHOL

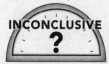

It's not unusual to find wines bearing the names of well-known people. ZinfandEllsbury, for example, is named for Boston Red Sox out-fielder Jacoby Ellsbury. Graceland Cellars offers up Velvet Elvis Cabernet Sauvignon. There's even a Palin Syrah—though blue-state sellers of this red wine insist that a resemblance to the name of any politician, living or dead, is purely coincidental.

Perhaps no one deserves his own vino more than Morley Safer. In 1991, the *60 Minutes* correspondent reported that red wine helped explain the so-called French Paradox—the fact that people in France have relatively low rates of heart disease despite their fatty, foie gras–filled diets. Safer's portrayal of red wine as a heart-healthy elixir caused sales to soar, and they've kept climbing. In 1991, red wine accounted for just 17 percent of the U.S. wine market, trailing far behind white wine. By 2009, red was the most popular type, with 47 percent of the market. Surely that calls for a Morley Merlot.

Whether Safer oversold the science is another matter. We have consistent evidence from numerous studies that moderate alcohol consumption (meaning one or two drinks a day) is associated with a lower risk of heart disease, diabetes, stroke, and premature death. But research is conflicting as to whether red wine is more beneficial than other forms of alcohol.

Red wine's alleged advantages are often attributed to an antioxidant called resveratrol, which is found in grape skins. (Because white wine is generally produced without the skins, it contains little if any resveratrol.) Studies in animals and test tubes suggest that the compound may have cardiovascular benefits, including relaxing blood vessels, preventing blood clots, and reducing inflammation. There's evidence that other substances in red wine, such as flavanols—which are in dark chocolate as well (see "Chocolate Is Good for You" on page 64)—may also be good for the heart.

But other research shows that alcohol itself may help the heart by increasing HDL (good) cholesterol and preventing blood clots. This raises the question of whether it's really the alcohol that explains any benefits of red wine.

Cohort studies don't provide clear answers. In some research, wine (both red and white) was associated with lower rates of heart disease and death, while the benefits of beer and hard liquor were smaller or nonexistent. In other studies, all moderate drinkers appeared to benefit equally, regardless of what type of alcohol they consumed.

Another consideration is that wine drinkers tend to smoke less and have more healthful diets than other imbibers, according to research. As a result, any apparent health advantages of red wine could be due to the drinkers rather than the drink.

One thing we know for certain is that binge or heavy drinking (meaning more than three drinks a day) is harmful. What's more, red wine isn't medicine, so you shouldn't feel compelled to drink it. Instead, go with what you most enjoy. If Palin wine isn't your cup of tea, for example, there's always Barbra Streisand Chardonnay. Personally, I'm sticking with my Roy Rogers.

Grape juice, like red wine, may benefit the heart by relaxing blood vessels, boosting good cholesterol, and preventing blood clots. But it's unknown whether drinking grape juice lowers rates of heart attacks, strokes, and premature death as red wine and other alcoholic beverages appear to do.

ALCOHOL CAUSES BREAST CANCER

If you're looking for ways to mark National Breast Cancer Awareness Month, going out drinking may not come immediately to mind. But some bars and liquor companies are trying to change that. Across the country, pubs and restaurants are hosting special events, sponsored by Chambord vodka, featuring pink cocktails. They're part of the company's Pink Your Drink campaign to raise awareness and money for breast cancer.

Likewise, the makers of Mike's Hard Lemonade sell a special pink version of their alcoholic beverage, with some of the proceeds going to breast cancer–related causes. On the company's website are comments from grateful patrons, such as "Thanks so much for making a big batch of pink lemonade to fight breast cancer!!"

You have to wonder whether these customers and the Pink Your Drink attendees are aware of a not-so-delicious irony: The beverages they're purchasing to fight breast cancer could in fact be causing it.

Over the past three decades, more than 100 case-control and cohort studies have examined the issue of alcohol consumption and breast cancer. As a whole, the research shows that women who consume at least a drink a day—whether beer, wine, or hard liquor—have slightly higher odds of developing breast cancer than those who abstain or have only an occasional drink. The more alcohol a woman consumes, the greater her risk.

Though scientists aren't entirely sure why, they suspect alcohol may make women more susceptible to breast cancer by raising levels of the hormone estrogen. Bolstering this theory is research showing that drinkers are more likely to have tumors that are hormone-receptor positive. Another proposed explanation is that alcohol depletes levels of certain nutrients that help protect against cancer.

Complicating matters is the fact that alcohol may also have health benefits. Many studies have linked it to lower odds of heart disease and stroke. How best to balance alcohol's Jekyll and Hyde sides depends on a woman's individual situation. For example, a woman in her 40s who's at increased risk of breast cancer because of family history or other factors may want to keep her alcohol intake to a minimum. On the other hand, for a woman in her 70s, when death rates due to heart disease far exceed those for breast cancer, the benefits of a daily glass or two of wine may outweigh any risks.

As a result, maybe those booze-fest fund-raisers for breast cancer should be targeted at wine-sipping grandmas. Or better yet, replace them with events that involve exercise, which is associated with a lower risk of the disease. I may not be able to attend, however. I'll be busy organizing a diabetes fund-raiser at my local doughnut shop.

Light and moderate drinkers have a lower risk of dementia and Alzheimer's disease than those who abstain. The evidence is strongest for wine drinkers.

YOU NEED EIGHT GLASSES OF WATER A DAY FOR GOOD HEALTH

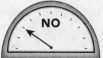 Which do you consider more important: sex or water?

No, it's not a question from one of those relationship-wrecking party games. It was actually the subject of a survey of 1,000 women, who were asked to prioritize various behaviors related to health and well-being. Surprisingly, respondents ranked "drinking the recommended amount of water" ahead of sex—as well as exercise.

It's a sign of how deeply ingrained the message has become that guzzling at least eight glasses of water a day is essential for good health. The list of purported benefits is lengthy—everything from smoothing skin to warding off cancer. But a look at the evidence shows that such claims, for the most part, are all wet.

Many people who constantly chug water will tell you they do so to get rid of toxins. That's the job of several organs, including the kidneys, and there's no evidence that lots of water helps improve their effectiveness. In fact, it's possible that extra H_2O may slightly *decrease* the kidneys' ability to filter out harmful substances.

Studies looking at the relationship between water consumption and bladder cancer have yielded inconsistent results. As for the effects on skin tone, one small study did find that drinking about two cups of water increased blood flow to the skin. But the researchers didn't assess whether this resulted in a smoother complexion. While it's true that being dehydrated may increase the appearance of fine lines, it doesn't follow that continuing to drink when you're adequately hydrated makes skin look better.

So how can you tell if you're adequately hydrated? Leaders of the chugalug club claim that most of us are a quart low and don't know it. But a panel of experts convened by the Institute of Medicine analyzed the science and concluded that we actually have a fairly foolproof system to alert us when we need fluids. It's called thirst. According to the panel, most healthy people get enough water through normal consumption of foods (which supply about 20 percent of our water) and beverages, including coffee, tea, and juice.

There are a few instances in which extra water may be beneficial. Studies show that drinking lots of fluids can help prevent kidney stones in people who have previously had them. It also may be a good idea to drink up if you live in a hot climate or engage in strenuous exercise. But don't overdo it. Participants in endurance sports like marathons who aren't elite athletes and who consume large amounts of water throughout the event can develop an abnormally low sodium level. The condition, called hyponatremia, is potentially fatal.

In general, though, there's nothing wrong with drinking lots of water if it makes you feel better or healthier. Just be prepared for those extra bathroom trips to interfere with the number one health priority from that survey of women: getting enough sleep.

Research suggests that drinking two cups of water before meals may help promote weight loss in middle-aged and older people by reducing hunger and calorie intake. Younger adults may not experience such benefits, however.

DIET SODA MAKES YOU FAT

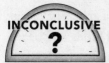

If you need evidence of just how much certain notions have changed in the last 50 years, try watching some old TV commercials. A classic example is a 1960s campaign for the diet soda Tab. With a sappy song and voiceover that seem straight out of a *Saturday Night Live* spoof, the commercials urge the female audience at whom they're targeted to "be a mind-sticker."

What the mad men behind this slogan meant was that women can remain in the thoughts of their absent (and presumably wandering-eyed) husbands by drinking Tab to stay slim and attractive. "A taste to remember," says one ad, "for a shape he can't forget."

Obviously, a blatantly sexist pitch like this would never fly today. Anyone who tried it would likely be boycotted out of business. Until recently, however, few people would have questioned the ad's premise that diet cola can help keep weight off. That's now starting to change as well because of media reports warning that drinking diet soda may actually *promote* obesity.

Such claims have arisen mainly from several cohort studies linking diet soda to weight gain and other risk factors for heart disease. In one study, which followed 3,700 people for seven to eight years, diet-soda drinkers who started out at normal weights were more likely to become overweight or obese than nondrinkers. The more they consumed, the more weight they gained.

Of course, this doesn't prove cause and effect. It's possible that as people start to put on pounds, they increase their intake of diet drinks.

Untangling all this requires intervention studies, and here the case loses some fizz. Such studies, in which an experimental group is fed sugar substitutes and compared to a control group, have generally failed to show that artificially sweetened foods and beverages cause weight gain. But the research hasn't conclusively demonstrated that they lead to weight loss either. Results are mixed, and some of the most frequently cited studies showing a benefit were funded by the artificial sweetener industry.

In short, it's unclear exactly how diet soda affects weight-control efforts. Still, scientists have several explanations as to why it may not help and could possibly hurt. One is the "I'll have a Big Mac, large fries, and a Diet Coke" fallacy: People may subconsciously (or consciously) assume that because they're being virtuous by drinking diet soda, it's okay to otherwise overindulge.

Another possibility is that artificial sweeteners mess with our minds. When we taste something sweet, our brains are alerted that calories are on the way. If they don't materialize because we're drinking an artificially sweetened beverage, we're driven to go seek them elsewhere. In such a way, diet sodas may prompt us to eat more.

If this turns out to be true, you might say diet soda is a "mind-sticker." Even after we're done, the drink continues to exert its influence on our brains. Somehow I doubt we'll be hearing about this in any ads.

Sports drinks are often wrongly perceived as a healthful alternative to soda for everyday use. Though they're lower in calories than regular soda, they can be relatively high in sugar. Plus, research shows they may erode tooth enamel more than soda does. The electrolytes in sports drinks can benefit people doing very strenuous exercise, but they're unnecessary for most of us.

JUICING IS THE BEST WAY TO GET NUTRIENTS

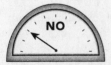

As a kid, I remember watching Jack LaLanne's TV show with my sister while we ate breakfast. Clad in his tight jumpsuit, the late fitness guru would often lecture viewers about the importance of proper nutrition. To us he seemed like a freak, and we'd laugh as we wolfed down our doughnuts and chocolate Pop-Tarts.

But I'm not laughing now. Remarkably healthy and energetic until his death at age 96, the man was clearly on to something. So what kind of diet did he recommend? For one thing, it included lots of fresh-squeezed juice from fruits and vegetables. LaLanne even had his own line of juicing machines, ads for which proclaimed "Jack LaLanne is living proof that juicing really works."

There's no question that juice is more nutritious than soda and, depending on the type of juice, a potentially good source of certain vitamins and minerals. Juicing can make it easier to meet your daily requirement of fruits and veggies. But talk to some enthusiasts, and you'll hear claims that a tall drink of dandelions and wheatgrass can increase energy, boost the immune system, and remove toxins. A common explanation is that because the digestive system doesn't have to break down food, the nutrients in juice are more easily absorbed, and the body is able to rest and heal itself.

Sounds good, but it's scientifically baseless. There's no evidence that juices are any more healthful or nutritious than the foods from which they come. Nor do we have proof that juicing promotes weight loss, as some claim. If you're not careful, it can have the opposite effect because certain juices are relatively high in calories. An eight-ounce glass of apple juice, for example, has 114 calories, compared to 97 in Coke. A concoction of several juices can contain even more calories.

Another possible pitfall is that juices from fruits and some veggies are loaded with the sugar fructose. Preliminary research suggests that large amounts may make the body resistant to insulin, and cohort studies have linked fruit juice consumption to an increased risk of diabetes.

Unlike juice, whole fruits and vegetables contain fiber, which helps the body process sugar more slowly and avoid the swings in blood sugar levels that you can get from juice. By drinking instead of eating your produce, you also miss out on the other possible health benefits of fiber and the feeling of fullness that it provides. What's more, you don't get the many healthful compounds found in the skin and pulp of fruits and vegetables.

If you enjoy juicing, go for it. But don't let it keep you from eating whole fruits and veggies. And despite what those ads imply, don't expect it to turn you into Jack LaLanne. For that you need to hit the gym—and lay off the doughnuts and Pop-Tarts.

Overall, orange juice is the most nutritious type of fruit juice, according to an analysis by the Center for Science in the Public Interest. One glass contains more than 100 percent of the daily requirement of vitamin C, and it's a good source of potassium and certain B vitamins. Grapefruit juice comes in second, but be careful because it can interact with certain medications. Apple juice ranks at the bottom in nutrients.

CRANBERRY JUICE PREVENTS URINARY INFECTIONS

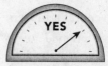

If you're a journalist long enough, you're bound to make at least a few enemies. Some reporters incur the wrath of political leaders. For others, it's celebrities, business executives, or mob bosses. In my glamorous work, it's cranberries—or, more precisely, the people who market them.

Years ago I wrote a newspaper column questioning some of the health claims made by cranberry producers. Their public relations firm—yes, like many other fruits, cranberries have a press agent—wrote an angry letter to the paper denouncing me and my reporting. I think of this every Thanksgiving as I dig into my meal and experience fleeting paranoia about someone poisoning my cranberry sauce to avenge the offending article.

Well, here's my chance to make amends: It turns out that the old folk remedy of drinking cranberry juice to prevent urinary infections has scientific merit.

In a review of 10 randomized trials, researchers concluded that cranberry juice and supplements reduce the frequency of urinary tract infections (UTIs) in women who get them repeatedly. One of the studies, which was conducted in Canada, involved 150 women with a history of UTIs. They were randomly assigned for a year to drink three glasses of cranberry juice a day, take cranberry pills, or get fake juice and fake pills. The juice drinkers and pill takers were less likely than the controls to get a UTI.

The reason, research suggests, is that cranberries contain substances called proanthocyanidins, which adhere to *E. coli* (the cause of the vast majority of UTIs) and prevent the bacteria from sticking to the bladder wall.

It's less clear whether cranberry juice can prevent UTIs in men, who are far less susceptible than women. There's no evidence it can treat infections once they occur.

Many people find pure cranberry juice unpalatable because it's so tart. Fortunately, cranberry juice cocktail, which has added sweeteners, also seems to work. But there's a drawback: The sugar-sweetened cocktail can be even higher in calories than soda.

Studies on UTIs and cranberry juice have varied in length

(everywhere from a month to a year), so it's unknown exactly how long you need to keep chugging to get a benefit. The same goes for the amount, though research suggests that the three glasses a day used in the Canadian study may be more than necessary.

One frequently mentioned concern is that cranberry juice can interact with the blood thinner warfarin (Coumadin) to increase the risk of bleeding. But a review of the research has concluded the danger is overstated and that up to 2.5 cups a day doesn't appear to pose a problem for people on the medication.

On that note, I think I'll stop. Now maybe the cranberry producers will remove me from their most-wanted list, and I can eat my next Thanksgiving meal in peace.

The substances in cranberry juice thought to prevent UTIs may also reduce the risk of stomach ulcers. Research suggests that cranberry juice can suppress *Helicobacter pylori*, the bacterium that causes most ulcers, and keep it from sticking to the intestinal wall.

GREEN TEA PROMOTES WEIGHT LOSS

Over the years, I've seen more questionable products for weight loss than I can count. Things like seaweed patches that allegedly boost your metabolism, rings for your finger that supposedly have the same effect as jogging six miles, and insoles for your shoes that purportedly prompt your body to burn fat.

Then there's green tea. The drink's reputation as a weight-loss aid took off after a diet book author claimed on *Oprah* that by simply switching from coffee to green tea, people could lose body fat "very rapidly" and shed 10 pounds in six weeks. When Coca-Cola and Nestlé tried to jump on the bandwagon with a beverage made of green tea extracts that would supposedly help burn extra calories, they were hit with an investigation by 28 states for making unsubstantiated claims. Eventually, they agreed to pay a fine and change their marketing to say that the drink, called Enviga, couldn't produce weight loss without dieting and exercise.

Given all the hype, green tea would seem to rank up there with diet rings and seaweed patches. In truth, it can really help burn extra calories—though probably not enough to make much of a difference.

Green tea contains an antioxidant known as epigallocatechin gallate (EGCG), which has been shown in lab studies to boost metabolism and fat burning. The caffeine in tea is thought to have similar effects. In a study of 10 men, the combination of EGCG and caffeine caused subjects to burn more energy over a 24-hour period than did caffeine alone or a placebo.

A number of small randomized trials have tested whether tea or supplements containing these ingredients can produce weight loss. When researchers pooled data from 13 such studies, they found that subjects taking EGCG plus caffeine, typically for three months, shed one to three pounds more than those getting a placebo. Such a small difference, the authors noted, is "not likely clinically relevant."

It's unknown whether you can lose more pounds over a longer period of time or whether the weight stays off. What's more, it's not clear exactly how much green tea you need to consume because studies have used various doses of EGCG and caffeine. The populations studied have varied as well, which means scientists aren't certain who is most likely to benefit.

Another unknown is the long-term safety of green tea supplements. In more than two dozen cases, they've been linked to liver damage, especially when taken on an empty stomach.

If you want to give green tea a try, your best bet is to stick with beverages instead of pills. While it may give your metabolism a small boost, don't count on it to put you in shape for swimsuit season. That's especially true if you prefer your tea in the form of Jamba Juice smoothies or Starbucks Frappuccinos, which can come loaded with more than 400 calories. Compared to that, you'd be better off with fat-burning insoles. At least they're calorie free—and they might make your shoes more comfortable.

Drinking black or green tea with meals can decrease iron absorption from food by 50 percent. But adding lemon to your tea may help counter this effect. That's because lemon is high in vitamin C, which enhances the absorption of iron.

Chapter 2

Fat Chance

BUTTER IS MORE HEALTHFUL THAN MARGARINE

 In *The Butter Battle Book*, Dr. Seuss's parable about the Cold War arms race, the Zooks and Yooks duke it out over whether to eat their bread with the butter side up or down.

In real life, there's a longstanding butter battle that has outlasted the Cold War. It involves not where butter goes but whether to use it. With apologies to Dr. Seuss, here's how butter lovers might describe the fight:

> *The spread on their bread, it's nothing but junk.*
> *It fills up their hearts with all kinds of gunk.*
> *Butter from cows is how we taste our toast.*
> *It keeps us alive and strong in the most.*

Twenty years ago, margarine supporters had the upper hand in the butter vs. margarine battle. But recently, butter has taken the lead, as many people have come to regard it as a more natural and healthful alternative to margarine. Whether butter is really better depends on what type of margarine you're comparing it to.

A big boost for butter came from the Nurses' Health Study, which involved more than 85,000 women. It found that those who ate four or more teaspoons of margarine a day had a higher risk of heart disease than those who used margarine only rarely. There was no increase in risk among butter eaters. A smaller cohort study of middle-aged men yielded similar findings.

These results came as a surprise to many. After all, margarine, which is made from vegetable oils, is lower in saturated fat than butter. But the process of converting those oils into solids can result in trans fats, which are thought to be even more hazardous to the heart than the saturated kind (see "Trans Fats Are Harmful" on page 31).

A study published in the *New England Journal of Medicine* seemed to further bolster the case for butter—to a point. Researchers had subjects eat various types of spreads and then measured the effects on cholesterol levels. Compared to butter, margarine lowered LDL (bad) cholesterol, but it also reduced HDL, the good kind. How much it lowered each—and hence the overall impact on heart health—varied according to the type of margarine. The big loser in this face-off was stick margarine, which fared worse than butter. Semiliquid margarine, on the other hand, proved to be *more* healthful than butter.

Since that research, manufacturers have introduced soft and

liquid margarines that are low in saturated fat and virtually free of trans fat. That makes them a better option than butter.

Still, some people refuse to touch any type of margarine because, unlike butter, it's not "natural." One widely circulated email message, for example, warns that margarine is just one molecule away from being plastic. "Would you melt your Tupperware and spread that on your toast?" the email asks.

While the plastic claim is silly (not to mention really unappetizing), margarine isn't exactly a health food. Nor is butter. Just as Dr. Seuss leaves his butter battle unresolved, there's no real winner here either. Your best bet is to minimize your use of both margarine and butter, going instead with healthful vegetable oils (such as olive or canola) whenever possible. Or as Dr. Seuss might have put it:

Do not spread them in a house.
Do not spread them with a mouse.
Do not spread them here or there.
Do not spread them anywhere.

Some margarines contain added compounds known as plant sterols and stanols, which have been shown to lower LDL (bad) cholesterol by up to 15 percent or more. To see an effect, you need at least two grams a day—the amount typically in two tablespoons of margarine. Some research suggests that getting the entire dose at once in the morning may not be effective, so it's best to use smaller amounts two or more times throughout the day.

OLIVE IS THE MOST
HEALTHFUL TYPE OF VEGETABLE OIL

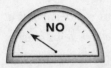

If the olive oil industry wanted a poster girl, it would have to be Jeanne Calment. The French-woman took up fencing at age 85, rode a bike until she was 100, and lived to be 122, earning the Guinness World Records title for the oldest person of all time whose age could be verified. (Tough luck, Methuselah.) She credited her youthfulness and longevity to olive oil, which she used liberally as not only a food but also a skin moisturizer.

Madame Calment wasn't the first olive oil apostle. In ancient Greece, the physician Hippocrates prescribed it for an array of ailments, and many people today regard it as the most healthful type of vegetable oil. While olive oil does appear to have health benefits, the claim that it's superior to all other oils is a bit slippery.

A key part of the so-called Mediterranean diet (see "A Mediterranean Diet Is Good for You" on page 137), olive oil is often singled out because it's high in monounsaturated fat. But it's also lower in polyunsaturated fat than other common cooking oils, like canola, safflower, and corn. Both monounsaturated and polyunsaturated fats are considered "good" fats that may reduce the risk of heart disease.

Which of these fats is better for us is unclear. Some research suggests that polyunsaturated fats may have an edge when it comes to lowering LDL (bad) cholesterol, while monounsaturated fats may result in higher HDL (good) cholesterol. A meta-analysis of 14 studies called it a draw, concluding that replacing saturated fat with either monounsaturated or polyunsaturated fat has an equally beneficial effect on cholesterol levels.

Another meta-analysis, this one of 11 cohort studies, went a step further, looking at heart attacks. And here the news wasn't good for monounsaturated fat: Substituting it for saturated fat was associated with an *increased* risk of heart attacks, while polyunsaturated fat was linked to lower odds.

While these results aren't necessarily an indictment of olive oil—the research lumped it in with other sources of monounsaturated fat, like animal fat, which could have different effects—they poke holes in the notion that its high levels of monounsaturated fat make olive oil more healthful.

Some people point to olive oil's lower levels of polyunsaturated fats as an advantage when it comes to cancer. In fact, there's some research linking certain kinds of polyunsaturated fats (specifically so-called omega-6 fatty acid, as opposed to omega-3 fatty acid found in fish) to breast, prostate, and other cancers. But overall, the findings are conflicting and far from conclusive.

Another theory is that antioxidants in olive oil known as polyphenols make it more healthful than its rivals. Research suggests that virgin and extra-virgin oils, which are high in polyphenols, may be more heart healthy than refined olive oil. But the evidence is preliminary and doesn't shed much light on how virgin oils stack up against non-olive oils.

The upshot of all this uncertainty is that other oils, such as canola, may be just as healthful as olive oil, if not more so. Of course, olive oil makers will continue trying to convince us otherwise. If they want to do so by invoking Jeanne Calment, they may have to line up behind cigarette companies. It turns out she was a smoker her entire adult life—until age 117. Now there's a record no one is likely to break anytime soon.

Extra virgin olive oil (or EVOO, as it's come to be known thanks to Rachael Ray) is extracted from the first pressing of olives, without chemicals or heat. It's the least processed type. *Pure* is a mixture of virgin and refined oil (derived from later pressing). *Light* refers to the color and flavor, not the number of calories.

FISH OIL PREVENTS HEART DISEASE

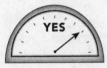

Through the years, I've come across all kinds of stories about inhabitants of exotic, far-away places who have reportedly eluded the ills plaguing modern civilization: They rarely get cancer. They're never depressed. They don't gain weight. They're free of arthritis, backaches, and foot fungus. They live to 150.

Typically, their robust health is attributed to something they eat or don't eat. In many cases, these dietary secrets—as well as the stories themselves—tend to fizzle under further scrutiny.

The tale of the Greenland Eskimos appears to be an exception. Decades ago, scientists discovered that the Inuit, as they're known, rarely died from heart disease despite a diet high in fat from fish. Researchers theorized that the fish fat was somehow protective— an idea that subsequent research has largely supported.

Several cohort studies show that regular fish eaters are less likely to die of heart disease than those who don't eat fish. Randomized trials involving heart attack survivors have found that subjects given fish oil supplements were less likely to die of heart disease than those who didn't take the capsules. And in a randomized study of people with and without heart disease who had high cholesterol, participants who took fish oil had fewer heart attacks and deaths from heart disease.

The key ingredients appear to be the omega-3 fatty acids eicosapentaenoic acid (EPA) and docosahexaenoic acid (DHA), which are found in most fish but especially oily ones such as salmon, mackerel, trout, sardines, and tuna. Studies suggest these fats may work their magic on the heart by relaxing blood vessels, reducing blood pressure, preventing abnormal rhythms, and lowering blood fats known as triglycerides.

While the evidence is strong for people who have heart disease or are at high risk for it, it's less clear whether fish oil wards off heart attacks in those at low risk. Still, it seems reasonable to follow the American Heart Association's recommendation and eat oily fish at least twice a week. People with heart disease are advised to get twice as much—the equivalent of 1,000 mg/day of EPA and DHA combined. To lower your triglycerides, you need 3,000 to 4,000 mg/day.

If the prospect of eating lots of salmon or sardines seems less than appetizing, there are always fish oil supplements. Just read labels carefully to make sure the pills contain adequate doses of EPA and DHA.

Krill oil, which comes from tiny, shrimp-like shellfish, is often promoted as a superior alternative to conventional fish oil supplements. Though the EPA and DHA from krill oil may be better absorbed, there's little evidence that it's more effective than fish oil.

The main side effect of conventional supplements is fishy burps. Think of it as the price we pay for trying to bottle and sell the Inuit's dietary secret. I can hear them laughing in their igloos.

Margarine, eggs, and other foods with added omega-3 fatty acids typically contain a form known as alpha-linolenic acid (ALA), which comes from plant sources such as flaxseed and canola oil rather than fish. The body converts ALA into DHA and EPA, but in fairly low amounts. The health benefits of ALA are not as well documented as those of fish oil.

EGGS ARE BAD FOR YOUR HEART

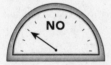

It's a *Time* magazine cover that's forever etched in my memory: a plate of eggs and bacon in the shape of a face, with the eggs serving as eyes and the bacon a frowning mouth. The headline on the article said it all: "Hold the Eggs and Butter; Cholesterol Is Proved Deadly, and Our Diets May Never Be the Same."

The year was 1984. As a college student with a budding interest in nutrition, I found the story so compelling that I vowed never to touch another egg (not too tough when your only option is runny scrambled eggs from the college cafeteria). I saved the article in a special file, believing that someday it would rank up there with "Men Walk on Moon" and other reports of history-making developments. Little did I know that this eggs-are-deadly story would really belong with the likes of "Titanic Sunk, No Lives Lost" and "Dewey Defeats Truman."

Since *Time*'s egg alarm, researchers have conducted a number of long-term cohort studies on eggs and heart disease, which have collectively followed several hundred thousand people. In general, the research has exonerated eggs: Eating up to six a week doesn't appear to be harmful for most healthy people.

So how can this be if egg yolks are high in cholesterol, and too much cholesterol is bad for us? Most of our cholesterol is made by the liver, which ramps up production when we eat saturated and trans fats. But cholesterol from food appears to have little impact on most people's cholesterol levels. And in people it does affect—so-called hyper-responders—studies show there can be an increase in good (HDL) cholesterol along with the bad kind (LDL), which helps offset any increased risk. Further, dietary cholesterol may also result in larger LDL particles, which are thought to pose less of a threat than smaller ones.

Eggs are relatively low in saturated fat, and they contain unsaturated fats, which may be beneficial. Plus, they're a good source of protein and several vitamins and minerals. They can be a healthful and more filling alternative to high-calorie muffins, bagels, and sugary cereals.

Before this starts sounding like an appeal from the egg industry to eat omelets with abandon, I should mention a few caveats: Some research has linked daily egg consumption to an increased risk of heart failure and type 2 diabetes. And several studies have found an association between eggs and heart disease, as well as premature death, among people who have diabetes. Scientists aren't sure why, but to be safe, it's probably a good idea for egg eaters with diabetes to watch their intake.

For most people, the biggest problem with eggs is what accompanies them. If your idea of an egg breakfast is IHOP's Big Steak Omelette or McDonald's Bacon, Egg, & Cheese Biscuit, that frowning face from 1984 still applies. To update it, just add puffy cheeks and extra-salty tears.

While yolks contain the cholesterol in eggs, they also contain most of the nutrients. The yolks and whites both contain protein.

NUTS PREVENT HEART ATTACKS

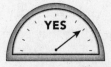 Some of us started talking earlier than others. For Mr. Peanut, the monocled mascot for Planters, it took 94 years. With a little help from actor Robert Downey Jr., the top hat–wearing, cane-wielding peanut uttered his first words in a TV ad in 2010.

It was part of an overhaul for Mr. Peanut (complete with the addition of a gray suit and bronze coloring), which was intended to make him—and the product he represents—more appealing.

Whatever its success, this image makeover can't top the one that the peanut (which technically isn't a nut but a legume) and its fellow nuts have already undergone in recent years. Once regarded as high-fat nutritional villains to be avoided at all costs, nuts are now touted as a health food that can ward off heart disease. And years of research suggest the notion isn't as nutty as it may seem.

The first solid evidence came from a cohort study of more than 30,000 Seventh-Day Adventists. Nut eaters—especially those who indulged five or more times a week—were less likely to suffer heart attacks or die from them than people who consumed nuts rarely or never. The results were greeted with skepticism, however, because Seventh-Day Adventists have atypical lifestyles: They don't drink or smoke and are often vegetarians. It was therefore unclear whether the findings applied to other people.

Three subsequent cohort studies, involving hundreds of thousands of people from different populations, have put that concern to rest. Regardless of gender, age, location, or occupation, people who eat nuts have consistently been shown to have lower odds of heart disease and heart-related deaths.

These findings are bolstered by results from clinical trials demonstrating that nuts lower LDL (bad) cholesterol levels. They also appear to decrease inflammation in arteries, which may contribute to heart attacks.

So which nuts are best for you? If you listen to producers of peanuts, walnuts, or almonds, each will tell you that its nut is superior because of some ingredient it contains. Walnuts, for example, are richest in ALA, an omega-3 fatty acid (see "Fish Oil Prevents Heart Disease" on page 23), and peanuts contain resveratrol, a substance also found in red wine (see "Red Wine Is the Most Beneficial Type of Alcohol" on page 3).

The truth is that it's impossible to say which is best because no one has done a head-to-head comparison. All nuts are relatively high in unsaturated fats, which are thought to be good for the heart. Macadamias, cashews, and Brazil nuts have more saturated fat than other nuts (and hence are not allowed by the FDA to carry heart-related health claims), but the difference is relatively small.

All nuts are fairly high in calories, so it's important to pay attention to portion sizes. About a handful a day is enough to reap health benefits and, according to research, doesn't cause weight gain. It may even promote weight loss by helping you feel full. But going nuts and overindulging can quickly lead to extra pounds.

Not to be outdone by a talking Mr. Peanut, pistachio manufacturers have enlisted as spokespeople Snooki Polizzi of the TV show *Jersey Shore* and disgraced former Illinois governor Rod Blagojevich. Sometimes silence is golden.

Like peanuts, peanut butter can be heart healthy, but watch out for added ingredients such as sugar and *fully* hydrogenated oil, which means saturated fat. (In contrast, *partially* hydrogenated oil equals trans fat. See "Saturated Fat Is Bad for Your Heart" below and "Trans Fats Are Harmful" on page 31.) Ideally, the only ingredient should be peanuts.

SATURATED FAT IS BAD FOR YOUR HEART

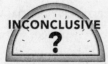

To make lessons stick with kids, you sometimes have to gross them out. Pictures of smokers' black, diseased lungs, for example, turned me off so much that I never touched a cigarette. Watching movies in driver's ed class of gruesome accidents ensured that I became a seat-belt wearer. And looking at vials containing gelatinous globs of fat, which represented what goes into your arteries when you eat burgers or butter, caused me to steer clear of saturated fat.

These graphic images are etched in my mind so vividly that I'll never forget the lessons they taught. But when it comes to fat, I may need to.

Leading sources of saturated fat include meat, whole dairy products, and lard. Experiments performed a century ago found that saturated fat can cause heart disease in animals. Early studies also showed it to raise cholesterol levels in people.

However, it was the work of scientist Ancel Keys that really put the issue of fat and heart disease on the map. Beginning in the 1950s, he observed that men in countries with the highest intake of saturated fat had the highest heart-related death rates, while populations with the lowest intake had the lowest death rates.

Keys's population studies were capable of showing only correlation, not cause and effect. To get more definitive evidence, scientists have performed dozens of additional studies over the decades. Surprisingly, despite all the dire warnings about the dangers of saturated fat, research as a whole has failed to prove that eating less of it reduces the risk of heart disease.

While some cohort studies have found a link between saturated fat and heart disease, many others have not. When researchers pooled data from 21 of these studies, they found no evidence of an association. Results from randomized trials have been similarly mixed.

One possible reason is that there are different types of saturated fat, which can have different effects. Certain kinds, such as stearic acid (which is found in high amounts in beef and chocolate), do not raise cholesterol levels. Others do, but they may boost HDL (good) cholesterol along with the bad kind (LDL), perhaps minimizing any harmful effects.

Another explanation for this big fat scientific mess is that when you eat less saturated fat, you eat more of something else—and not all substitutions are the same. Clinical trials show that replacing saturated with polyunsaturated fats, such as those found in nuts, fish, and vegetable oils (like safflower or corn oil), reduces the risk of heart disease. But swapping saturated fats for refined carbohydrates like low-fat cookies or white bread may not be any better for your heart and could even be worse, according to research. Trans fats are an especially bad alternative (see "Trans Fats Are Harmful" below).

All this complicates my mental imagery of saturated fat. Now when I think of that tube of goo, I also need to picture a vial of SnackWell's cookies alongside it. But I'm afraid that won't have quite the same impact. Instead of being grossed out, I'll just be hungry.

Palm and coconut oils contain a higher percentage of saturated fat than lard does. As a result, these oils have long been regarded as unhealthful. However, some newer studies suggest that they may not adversely affect cholesterol levels and may even have a beneficial effect.

TRANS FATS ARE HARMFUL

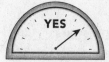

In my early 20s, I spent a summer interning for a consumer health group. One of my assignments was to create and display signs near a McDonald's restaurant protesting the unhealthfulness of their

food. While picketing is not exactly my thing, it beat stuffing enve-
lopes. Plus, I reasoned, I could raise awareness of a troubling but
little-known fact about McDonald's fries: They were cooked in
artery-clogging beef fat.

Thanks to complaints like this, McDonald's and other fast-
food restaurants eventually succumbed and switched to vegetable
oil. While my fellow protesters patted themselves on the back for
the victory, there was one not-so-little problem: The vegetable oil
used for frying contained partially hydrogenated (or trans) fat,
which it turned out is worse for you than beef fat. Oops.

Partially hydrogenated fats are created through a chemical
process that makes vegetable oils solid at room temperature. These
fats also occur naturally in small amounts in meat and dairy products. Because they help enhance creaminess, taste, and shelf life,
manufacturers have used them in an array of packaged foods, from
cookies and chips to margarines and peanut butter. The fact that
they can be used repeatedly makes them ideal for frying in restaurants.

Until the 1990s, there was a widespread perception that partially hydrogenated fats were a more healthful alternative to butter, beef fat, and palm and coconut oils, all of which are high in
saturated fat. But then research started to emerge suggesting otherwise. Like saturated fats, trans fats were found to raise LDL
(bad) cholesterol. But they also lowered HDL (good) cholesterol—
a double whammy.

Several cohort studies have found that people who consume
the most trans fats are more likely to develop heart disease. The
increased risk appears to come from artificially created trans fats,

not those that occur naturally in milk and meat. When researchers pooled results from four cohort studies, they concluded that even small amounts might pose a risk.

Scientists suspect that trans fats cause harm by not only affecting cholesterol levels but also raising blood fats called triglycerides, promoting inflammation in arteries, and adversely affecting the lining of blood vessels. Overall, the evidence suggests trans fats are more harmful than saturated fats, and it's more consistent.

As more places in the United States ban trans fats in restaurants, the food industry is working feverishly to develop new alternatives. Let's hope that these, unlike the previous "improvement," will prove safe in the long run. That way, protesters can direct their outrage at other burning issues, like the interminable wait at drive-through windows. I may even join in on that one.

On food labels, anything less than 0.5 gram of trans fat can legally be rounded down to zero. That means if you eat several servings of a so-called trans fat–free food—or a few such foods a day—you can wind up consuming measurable amounts of trans fat. To avoid it, check ingredient labels and steer clear of anything containing partially hydrogenated oils.

Chapter 3

Carb Games

CARBS MAKE YOU GAIN WEIGHT

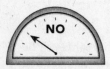 Of all the starchy foods blacklisted by low-carb diets, none has been vilified more than potatoes. When the federal government banned low-income women from buying white potatoes with food vouchers, it was the last straw for Chris Voigt. As head of the Washington State Potato Commission, he decided to take action. For two months, the man ate nothing but potatoes, consuming 20 a day in just about every form imaginable (though he skipped the butter and sour cream). In the end, he lost 21 pounds.

Commissioner Potato Head's publicity stunt, which made national headlines, didn't succeed in reversing the federal government's potato policy. But it did demonstrate a scientific truth more vividly than any study could: Carbohydrates aren't the main cause of weight gain, and you don't have to shun them to shed pounds.

Despite all the complicated explanations offered by various diet plans, weight comes down to simple math. If you take in more calories than you burn, you gain weight. If you consume fewer, you lose weight. In general, it doesn't matter whether those calories come from carbs, fat, or protein.

Support for this idea comes from more than a dozen randomized trials that have compared various types of diets. Though some show that low-carb diets result in greater weight loss during the first six months, any advantages disappear after one year.

In a longer-term study published in the *New England Journal of Medicine*, 800 overweight adults were randomly assigned to one of four diets, each with a different percentage of carbs, fat, and protein. Calories were also restricted. After two years, all four groups had lost the same amount of weight—about nine pounds on average.

Likewise, in a two-year randomized study that pitted a low-carb diet against a low-fat diet, the low-carb eaters lost no more weight. However, they did have a greater increase in their HDL (good) cholesterol levels. On the other hand, they were more likely to experience side effects such as bad breath, hair loss, constipation, and dry mouth.

Many low-carbohydrate diets have particular disdain for carbs like baked potatoes that have a high glycemic index (GI), which is an indicator of how rapidly a food causes blood sugar to rise. (A related measure, glycemic load [GL], takes into account both GI and the amount of carbohydrate per serving.) The theory is that keeping blood sugar levels consistently low promotes weight loss by causing the body to burn more fat and reducing hunger.

However, evidence for this idea is limited. Most weight-loss trials comparing GI or GL diets to other types have been small and short term, and they've produced conflicting results. One reason may be that the effects of a particular food on blood sugar can vary from person to person and from one instance to another depending in part on what else we're eating.

Chris Voigt's potato binge—which included consuming a mashed-up concoction molded into a turkey for Thanksgiving as he watched his family enjoy a large feast—resulted in an overall *drop* in his fasting blood sugar level as well as his cholesterol. No word on how it affected his sanity.

Ounce for ounce, white potatoes and sweet potatoes contain about the same number of calories. While white potatoes are higher in potassium, sweet potatoes have more fiber and vitamin C. Plus, they contain large amounts of vitamin A; a medium sweet potato provides more than seven times the daily requirement.

CARBS HELP YOU LOSE WEIGHT

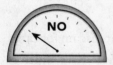

When I first heard a reference to "morning banana," I assumed it was the name of some wacky drive-time deejay. Well, I was right about the wacky part. It's actually a weight-loss diet that involves eating only bananas in the morning, followed by whatever you want for lunch or dinner. After a singer in Japan claimed that she'd lost 15 pounds on the regimen, sales of the fruit surged so much in that country that it experienced a banana shortage.

Proponents say a key component of this diet is something called resistant starch (RS), so named because it resists being broken down and absorbed as it passes through the small intestine. RS is found in not only bananas (especially green ones) but also foods such as potatoes, bread, and pasta—things that get the ax from Atkins and other low-carb diets. But these are the star attraction in weight-loss plans like the Skinny Carbs Diet and the Carb-Lovers Diet, which claim that RS can help you shed pounds by burning fat and reducing hunger. While preliminary studies seem to provide a bit of support for the idea, I wouldn't go bananas over it.

How foods are processed and cooked affects how much RS they contain. High on the list are unprocessed whole grains, corn flakes, uncooked rolled oats, white beans, cold pasta, raw potatoes, and cooked potatoes that have been cooled. RS also comes in the form of specially formulated cornstarch that can be sprinkled into foods or used as a substitute for flour.

Lab studies have found that feeding rodents a high RS diet results in less body fat, perhaps by increasing levels of hormones that make the animals feel full and stop eating. Advocates of RS diets often point to that research along with a human study in which subjects were fed four meals with varying amounts of RS. The meal containing about 5 percent RS (as a fraction of total carbs) resulted in 23 percent more fat burning than the one with no RS. Sounds impressive until you know a few details: The study consisted of just 12 subjects, they ate just one of each meal, and testing lasted for just 24 hours.

In general, human studies—all of them small and short term—

have yielded mixed results. Some show that RS increases feelings of fullness or results in lower food intake, but other research has found no such effects. There's little if any direct evidence that eating RS leads to weight loss, even in the short run.

If high RS diets do help you shed pounds, it may be because many RS foods are rich in fiber, which has been linked to lower body weight. In any event, you can't go wrong with oats, beans, brown rice, and other RS foods that are part of a healthful diet. But I'll skip the green morning bananas, thanks.

While there's no proof that eating bananas (at any time of day) will melt away pounds, there's also little evidence that they're especially fattening, as some diet plans claim. A medium banana has 105 calories, compared to 95 in a medium apple. Bananas are a good source of potassium, vitamin C, and fiber.

MULTIGRAIN FOODS ARE GOOD FOR YOU

HALF TRUE

The menu at Starbucks is a study in doublespeak. If you ask for a small, you get a tall, which is really a medium. A medium is a grande. A short is a small.

For college English teacher Lynne Rosenthal, this was irritating enough. But her attempt to order a plain multigrain bagel really sent her over the edge. When the barista at a Manhattan Starbucks asked if she wanted cream cheese or butter with her bagel, Rosenthal refused to answer, deeming it a superfluous question because she had asked for her bagel plain. A heated exchange ensued, with the professor becoming so worked up that the employees called the cops, who kicked her out of the place.

"Linguistically, it's stupid," she was quoted as saying about having to specify what she didn't want on a plain multigrain bagel. "I'm a stickler for correct English."

Maybe she should have saved her ire for the misleading use of the word *multigrain*. In some cases, multigrain foods may be healthful; but in others, they're no better for you than white bread.

A growing array of products—from bread and pasta to cookies and crackers—now proudly proclaim themselves to be multigrain. Many consumers assume the label is a synonym for *whole grain* or *whole wheat*. But it's not. It simply means the food is made from several grains, which may be refined.

In their natural state, grains consist of three parts: bran, germ, and endosperm. When they're refined to make white bread or pasta, the bran and germ are stripped away, leaving only the endosperm. This results in fewer nutrients and less fiber. Some nutrients are added back, which is why you often see the term *enriched* flour. But it's still refined.

Whole grains, in contrast, retain all parts of the grain. Examples include 100 percent whole wheat bread and pasta, brown rice, and oats, as well as less familiar varieties such as bulgur. Cohort studies have linked a diet rich in whole grains to a reduced risk of heart disease and diabetes. Whole grains can also help prevent constipation and other digestive problems.

Multigrain foods don't necessarily have such benefits because they may contain few, if any, whole grains. Consider, for example, multigrain Pringles potato chips. The canister and TV ads for the product prominently feature stalks of wheat, giving the impression that the chips are whole wheat. Yet the main ingredient is actually rice flour (which is refined), along with a smattering of wheat bran, barley flour, and dried black beans. The fiber content—a measly one gram per serving—is no greater than what you get in regular Pringles.

To avoid falling for marketing tricks like this, beware of not only the term *multigrain* but also descriptors such as *12 grain* (or any other number) and *made with whole grains*. Also, don't assume something is whole grain just because it's brown or involves wheat somehow. Instead, check the ingredients to make sure the first one listed contains the word *whole*.

That's not the case with the Starbucks multigrain bagel that prompted the professor's meltdown. The main ingredient is refined flour. But I wouldn't suggest picking a fight over it with the barista. Just order the fruit cup instead.

Sprouted-grain breads are often touted as nutritionally superior to other breads. Although they can sometimes have slightly higher amounts of protein and certain nutrients, there's little evidence that they're more healthful than conventional whole-grain breads.

OATS LOWER CHOLESTEROL

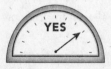

Mention the excesses of the 1980s, and most people think of finance or fashion. For me, the first thing that comes to mind is . . . oat bran. For those too young to remember (or too normal to share my fixation on such matters), oat bran was all the rage in the late '80s because of its purported power to lower cholesterol. After a 1987 bestselling book titled *The 8-Week Cholesterol Cure* hailed oat bran as a magic bullet, the stuff started popping up in everything from muffins to breads to potato chips. Sales of Quaker Oats oat bran cereal reportedly rose 20-fold between 1987 and 1989.

The frenzy ended in 1990, when a study published in the *New England Journal of Medicine* cast doubt on the effectiveness of oat bran. The bran retreated back into relative obscurity, but oats didn't.

A few years later, the FDA gave its blessing for claims on oatmeal, Cheerios, and other foods that oats can reduce the risk of heart disease by reducing cholesterol. But then in 2009, the agency ordered the makers of Cheerios to stop saying that the cereal could lower cholesterol.

It's understandable if all these zigzags have left you feeling dizzy. Fortunately, the science tells a less complicated story: There's decent evidence that whole oats—whether in oatmeal, oat cereal, or oat bran—are beneficial.

Oats contain a type of soluble fiber known as beta-glucan, which is also found in barley. It's thought to lower cholesterol by binding to bile acids and removing them from the body. Bile acids are made from cholesterol, so when the body has to deploy more of its cholesterol to help replace the eliminated bile acids, there's less of it in the blood. Essentially, cholesterol is forced to work, so it won't hang out and cause mischief.

The Cochrane Collaboration, an independent group that assesses the evidence for various treatments, conducted a meta-analysis of eight randomized studies involving people with elevated cholesterol and other risk factors for heart disease. Subjects assigned to eat oat cereal every day lowered their total and LDL (bad) cholesterol levels seven or eight points more than those on a diet of refined grains. Oats did not appear to affect HDL (good) cholesterol, however.

The studies lasted only four to eight weeks, so we don't know about long-term effects. What's more, much of the research was funded by food companies that sell oat products. Nevertheless, the science as a whole suggests that the effects are real.

To see a benefit, you need three grams of beta-glucan a day, which you can get from 1.5 cups of cooked oatmeal, 3 cups of instant oatmeal, or 3 cups of Cheerios. Which raises the question: If the oats in Cheerios lower cholesterol, why did the FDA clamp down on the claims? The problem was the wording, which violated FDA rules because it made the cereal sound like a medication.

Certainly, oats are not a wonder drug, and they need to be combined with a heart-healthy diet and exercise. Also, just not any oat product will do. Unfortunately, oatmeal cookies and Chocolate Cheerios (which are higher in sugar than in oats) don't count.

Research suggests that oat beverages are even more effective than cereals at lowering cholesterol. Just wait until food manufacturers get wind of this. Before long, we may have an oat juice craze on our hands. If so, I'll definitely be sitting that one out.

Instant oatmeal has as much soluble fiber as slower-cooking varieties of oats, such as old-fashioned and steel-cut.

GLUTEN IS HARMFUL

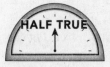 I have an unusual food addiction: I'm a whole-wheat junkie. Put a loaf of wheat bread in front of me, and I typically devour it in one sitting. Whether it's bagels, cereal, pasta, or pizza dough, I rarely meet a wheat product I don't love. I'm even a fan of those low-salt, fat-free, whole-wheat crackers, whose taste some of my friends and family liken to cardboard. (Not that they know what cardboard tastes like. Or maybe they do.)

For me to give up wheat, my life would have to depend on it. For some people, though, that's literally the case. They suffer from celiac disease, a condition in which eating gluten—a protein in wheat, barley, and rye—damages the lining of the small intestine, impairing the body's ability to absorb nutrients. The possible effects include gastrointestinal problems, anemia, rashes, infertility, and weakened bones, among other things.

The condition, which is diagnosed with a blood test and biopsy, is estimated to affect a bit less than 1 percent of the population. The only way to control it and reverse the symptoms is to adopt a gluten-free diet, which entails avoiding everything from beer and bologna to pasta and waffles.

The case against gluten isn't nearly as clear-cut for the other 99 percent of people, but a growing number are nevertheless forgoing the protein. Some say they have trouble digesting it (similar to the way many people can't handle lactose, the sugar in milk) and that avoiding foods containing gluten makes them feel better. Since there's no established medical test for this non-celiac form of gluten intolerance, we have to take their word for it.

There's less reason to believe claims that a gluten-free diet can fight a wide array of medical conditions, from arthritis to diabetes. One of the most frequently mentioned is autism. Though some research has hinted that autistic children who avoid gluten may show slight improvements, it's far too preliminary to warrant any firm conclusions.

Celebrities like Elisabeth Hasselbeck, cohost of *The View*, go even further, promoting the notion that shunning gluten can enhance everyone's overall health. Hasselbeck, who has celiac disease and has authored a book about what she calls the "G-Free" diet, writes that it "can help with weight management . . . elevate your energy levels, improve your attention span, and speed up your digestion" even if you don't have celiac disease or gluten intolerance. Maybe a better name would have been "E-Free," with the *E* standing for *evidence*.

Still, a gluten-free diet may be beneficial if it forces you to cut back on refined carbohydrates like pastries, cookies, and white bread, as well as calories overall. But if you simply replace such foods with the growing number of gluten-free packaged products, you could wind up worse off because they can be higher in sugar and calories. These foods also tend to be lower in fiber and B vitamins, and cost significantly more than their gluten-containing counterparts.

Because of the ubiquity of gluten in foods, avoiding it requires considerable effort. I prefer to spend my time scouring supermarkets for cardboard-flavored crackers.

Quinoa, an increasingly popular gluten-free food, is widely considered a whole grain. Technically, it's not; it's the seed of a plant related to spinach. But like whole grains, quinoa is high in fiber.

FIBER PREVENTS COLORECTAL CANCER

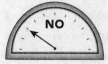 If you think your job is crappy, consider the work of Dr. Denis Burkitt. He spent his time analyzing feces. He weighed it, observed its odor and texture, and recorded how frequently people produced it.

No, this wasn't some kind of weird fetish. Burkitt, a British surgeon working in Africa, observed that colorectal cancer and various other conditions—including heart disease, diabetes, hemorrhoids, and constipation—were relatively rare among Africans. He concluded that the reason was the high levels of fiber in their diets, which resulted in large, soft stools and frequent bowel movements. He set out to prove his theory and popularized it in a best-selling book.

Burkitt's pioneering work spawned lots of further research on dietary fiber and colorectal cancer, including several dozen case-control studies. The vast majority seemed to support his hypothesis that high fiber results in a lower risk.

The findings were bolstered by plausible scientific explanations: By increasing the amount of water in stool, researchers theorized, fiber dilutes cancer-causing substances. It also speeds up the movement of stool, reducing the time that cancer-causing substances sit in the colon.

But cohort studies, some of which followed hundreds of thousands of people for many years, tell a different story. While a few have linked high fiber intake to a lower risk of colorectal cancer, most have shown no association.

Randomized trials have also produced disappointing results. In one study, published in the *New England Journal of Medicine*, researchers assigned more than 2,000 people with a history of precancerous growths in the colon, known as polyps, to eat either a high-fiber diet or their normal fare. After four years, the fiber eaters had no fewer polyps. Another randomized study, following subjects for eight years, yielded similar results.

It's possible that the randomized and cohort studies failed to find anything because the amount of fiber in the high-fiber diets—typically about half or two thirds of the amount consumed by the Africans in Burkitt's studies—was not high enough. Or maybe subjects ate the wrong form of fiber. Bran cereal, for example, may have a different effect than fruits and vegetables.

Then again, it may simply be that Burkitt was wrong about fiber and colorectal cancer. However, we do have relatively consistent evidence that high-fiber diets protect against other gastrointestinal problems, including constipation and diverticulosis as well as heart disease and diabetes. Eating lots of fiber has also been associated with a lower risk of premature death.

So even if fiber doesn't ward off colorectal cancer, it's still a good idea to load up on high-fiber foods, including whole grains, fruits, veggies, beans, nuts, and seeds. And when all that fiber sends you to the bathroom, you can thank Dr. Burkitt.

Some packaged foods contain added fiber with names such as inulin, maltodextrin, and polydextrose. Though these count toward a food's fiber total, they may not have the same health benefits as the naturally occurring fiber found in fruits, vegetables, and whole grains. Plus, inulin can cause gastrointestinal discomfort.

Chapter 4

Sugar and Spice

HIGH-FRUCTOSE CORN SYRUP IS WORSE FOR YOU THAN SUGAR

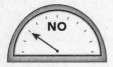

Whatever you think of high-fructose corn syrup (HFCS), you have to feel at least a little sympathy for the hapless souls assigned the task of boosting the sweetener's rotten image. When they conducted a $30 million advertising campaign intended to allay fears about the product's safety, the main result was a slew of parodies that mercilessly mocked the ads' message.

For example, in one real commercial, a woman questions a fellow mom for serving kids an HFCS-sweetened beverage. Confidently explaining that the product is "natural" and "fine in moderation," the HFCS user puts the accuser in her place and leaves her speechless. A series of YouTube spoofs shows two women engaged in a virtually identical conversation, except that the woman being questioned (played by a guy in drag) is defending lead-containing products from China, female genital mutilation, and KKK cross burnings.

You definitely have a PR problem when your product is likened to such things.

Food manufacturers, which use HFCS in everything from cereals to soda, like the sweetener because it's cheaper than sugar and prolongs the shelf life of products. But many people regard it as a sinister chemical concoction that's causing obesity along with diabetes, heart disease, and other conditions.

Indeed, lab experiments have found that rodents fed HFCS gained more weight than those receiving table sugar. The rats also showed signs of so-called metabolic syndrome—a combination of several risk factors, such as belly fat and increased blood pressure—which has been linked to heart disease and diabetes.

But there's little evidence from human studies that HFCS is any worse for our waistlines or our health than table sugar (also known as sucrose). The fact that HFCS and table sugar have a very similar chemical makeup also casts doubt on the claims. Both contain the sugars fructose (the type in fruit) and glucose in roughly equal proportions. Moreover, HFCS has the same number of calories as table sugar.

One difference is that the fructose and glucose are chemically bonded in table sugar but not in HFCS. Some argue that as a result, our bodies metabolize table sugar and HFCS differently. At this point, however, it's just a theory with no hard proof.

We do have evidence that the body processes pure fructose differently than glucose. Broken down in the liver, fructose is more likely than glucose to result in the production of harmful fats.

There are also hints that large amounts of fructose may make the body resistant to insulin. Whether the cumulative amount we get from HFCS actually causes harm is unknown.

The fact that HFCS is processed (and not "natural," as those industry ads have claimed) doesn't necessarily render it a health risk, as some maintain. But even though the science to date hasn't proven HFCS to be uniquely villainous, the product isn't totally benign either. Like table sugar, it's a source of empty calories, and consuming too much sugar—in whatever form—can lead to obesity and related health problems.

In another effort to improve their product's image, the producers of HFCS are pushing to officially rename it "corn sugar." Getting a new identity has certainly worked for other foods, including canola oil (formerly rapeseed oil) and orange roughy (slimehead). I just wish Chinese restaurants could find a more appetizing name for the poo-poo platter.

Added sugar in processed foods can come in many forms besides HFCS, including brown rice syrup, evaporated cane juice, fruit juice concentrate, molasses, and agave nectar. Though these may sound more healthful than sugar or HFCS, there's no evidence that they are.

HONEY IS MORE HEALTHFUL THAN SUGAR

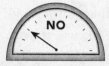

If you've ever wondered what a cross between a lobster and a blowfish looks like, you can find out by seeing me when I get stung by bees. It's not pretty. As a result, I try to stay as far away from them as I can. But a growing number of people apparently don't feel a similar need. Backyard beekeeping is booming, thanks in part to the grow-your-own-food movement. More people are drawn to the idea of producing their own honey, which according to one blogger, "has long been considered healthier than sugar."

At least that's the buzz. But the truth isn't quite so sweet for honey.

Honey is composed mainly of fructose and glucose, the same ingredients in table sugar (also known as sucrose). Some claim that our bodies respond more favorably to honey than to sugar, but there's little solid evidence for this.

On the glycemic index, which is a measure of how foods affect blood sugar levels, some types of honey cause less of a spike than sucrose, but generally both score about the same. Honey has come out ahead of sucrose in a few short-term studies comparing their effects on blood sugar, insulin levels, and cholesterol. However, the studies are too small and preliminary to tell whether these advantages are real or whether they translate into any lasting impact on people's health.

Another frequently cited advantage of honey is its higher levels of nutrients. Indeed, it does contain a number of vitamins and minerals not found in table sugar, including calcium, potassium, zinc, vitamin C, and niacin. However, the amounts are minuscule. To meet your daily requirement of calcium, for example, you would need 1,000 tablespoons of honey.

While antioxidant levels in honey vary depending on the plant source of the bees' nectar, one study found that overall, the antioxidant content of honey is higher than that of white sugar but lower than that of brown sugar. Whether these differences affect our risk of heart disease, cancer, or other conditions is unknown.

As for calories, honey actually has more than sugar—64 vs. 49 per tablespoon. But because honey is sweeter, you may need to use less.

Some people choose honey over sugar because they believe honey is less processed. In fact, typical store brands are processed with heat and filtration to remove wax, pollen, and other impurities. The alternative is raw honey, which enthusiasts swear is more healthful than processed honey. But here too the evidence is skimpy.

On a less sour note, honey isn't any worse for you than table sugar, and it can be a great addition to many foods and beverages. Just watch your intake as you would with sugar. If you want to become a beekeeper and produce your own honey, more power to you. All I ask is that you keep your bees far from me.

Research shows that honey, when applied to mild to moderate burns, can result in speedier healing than conventional dressings.

ASPARTAME IS UNSAFE

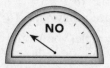

For journalists, press releases are a little like reality TV shows: They're totally unavoidable, mostly forgettable, and occasionally entertaining. One of my favorite releases came in 1998 during the Bill Clinton–Monica Lewinsky scandal. Titled "The Deposition of

President Clinton," it pointed out that when the former president underwent grand jury questioning about his relationship with Lewinsky, he repeatedly responded with answers like "My memory is not clear" and "I don't remember."

The release's author, a physician, noted that the president was drinking Diet Coke during the deposition. His conclusion: Aspartame (aka Equal and NutraSweet), the artificial sweetener in the beverage, was the cause of Clinton's apparent memory lapses.

Never mind that President Clinton's memory is otherwise extraordinary. The doctor, it turns out, is a longtime anti-aspartame crusader who was seeking to exploit the scandal for his cause. If nothing else, he deserves credit for knowing how to get attention— or at least a good laugh.

On the Internet you can find plenty of others who rail against aspartame for causing not only memory loss and Alzheimer's disease but also brain tumors, multiple sclerosis, depression, chronic fatigue syndrome, and birth defects, among other maladies. But decades of research have turned up little hard evidence for such assertions.

Though Italian researchers have found elevated rates of lymphoma, leukemia, and other cancers in rodents ingesting aspartame, most other animal studies have shown no connection between aspartame and cancer. More important, in a cohort study involving nearly 500,000 people, there was no increased risk of blood or brain cancers among aspartame users.

Likewise, most studies looking at neurological and behavioral issues haven't found adverse effects from aspartame. When a panel of scientists reviewed more than 500 studies, they uncovered no major safety problems. The review was funded by a Japanese manufacturer of aspartame, but the experts were unaware of who the funder was, and the company had no role in selecting the experts.

The panel's conclusions echo those of both the FDA and the European Commission's Scientific Committee on Food, which say that a daily intake of up to 40 or 50 milligrams of aspartame per kilogram of body weight is safe for most people. Translated into plain English, this means a 150-pound adult can safely consume up to about 19 cans of diet soda a day. (Not that anyone says drinking this much is advisable.) Obviously, most of us fall well below that threshold.

Still, aspartame may adversely affect certain people. One of the most common complaints is headaches, an effect detected by some (but not all) research. Also, people with a rare inherited condition called phenylketonuria (PKU) can't metabolize phenylalanine, an amino acid in aspartame. To avoid an unsafe buildup, they need to steer clear of the sweetener. (Hence that cryptic warning "Phenylketonurics: Contains Phenylalanine" on the labels of foods and beverages that contain aspartame.)

Despite the claims of some aspartame opponents, there's no solid proof that phenylalanine from normal amounts of aspartame poses a danger to the rest of us. The same goes for methanol, which is also produced when our bodies break down aspartame. In fact, we get more methanol from fruit juice than from aspartame.

Those who are convinced aspartame is poison or an evil plot may denounce me as an ignoramus or a pawn of industry for not agreeing with them. But at least they won't be able to blame my "confusion" on aspartame-related brain problems. Personally, I can't stand the taste.

Despite their name, sweeteners known as sugar alcohols, which are in sugarless gum, breath mints, toothpastes, and many foods, do not contain sugar or alcohol. They're often identifiable on labels by their "ol" endings (for example, lactitol, erythritol, maltitol, sorbitol, xylitol). They have fewer calories than sugar and don't raise blood sugar as much. However, some can cause gas, bloating, and diarrhea.

SEA SALT IS MORE HEALTHFUL THAN REGULAR SALT

It's amazing what one little word can do. The term *sea* when added to certain words with negative connotations has the power to make them positive. Take, for example, *weed*. Alone, it's a big nuisance in your yard, but pair it with *sea*, and you get a delicacy on your dinner plate. Even the word *dead*, which is about as negative as they come, gets an image makeover from *sea*, becoming one of the world's great tourist attractions.

Enter *salt*. From a health standpoint, it's a dirty word because it can raise blood pressure. Health authorities advise us to eat less of it. But as marketers are well aware, *salt* sounds much more benign when combined with *sea*, conjuring up images of gentle waves of sparkling, blue water lapping up on sandy, white beaches. Stick *natural* in front of *sea salt*, as many brands now do, and you've got a full-fledged health food. Or so it would seem.

Like table salt, sea salt is composed mainly of sodium and

chloride. Produced by the evaporation of seawater, it may also include trace amounts of other minerals from the water, such as magnesium, copper, and calcium.

In contrast, table salt is mined from underground salt deposits. During processing, trace minerals are removed and iodine is added, along with ingredients to prevent clumping.

While some people prefer cooking with sea salt because of its variety of textures and colors, as well as what they perceive to be a better taste, it offers no clear health advantage over table salt. By weight, both types contain about the same amount of sodium, which is what poses a health risk.

It's true that sea salt can come in lower-sodium varieties. (They're used in some store-bought soups, for example.) But there's nothing unique about this. You can also find reduced-sodium table salt.

Some claim that because sea salt is less processed, its sodium is somehow less harmful. But there's no solid evidence for this. Ditto for claims that the additional minerals provide a health boost. The levels are so low that they pack very little nutritional punch. However, the minerals can add extra flavor, which may let you go easier on the salt shaker.

One potential disadvantage of sea salt is that, unlike regular salt, it doesn't have added iodine. But for most Americans, this isn't a big problem. Manufacturers in the United States began putting the mineral in table salt in the 1920s because iodine deficiency was leading to high rates of goiter—an enlarged thyroid gland—in certain areas of the country. Today, it's easier to get adequate iodine through a normal diet that includes fish, dairy products, and plants from iodine-rich soil.

It's perfectly fine to use sea salt if you prefer it. Just take any implied health claims with a grain of salt. Personally, descriptors such as "from the blue waters of the Mediterranean Sea" or "made naturally from the sea and the sun" don't entice me to buy sea salt, but they definitely leave me hungering for a vacation.

Kosher salt contains less sodium *by volume* than table salt because it has much coarser grains that occupy more space. The same is true of some coarsely grained sea salts. But by weight, all have about the same sodium levels.

MSG IS HARMFUL

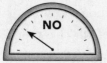

It's not every day that food manufacturers get into a full-fledged food fight. But that's what happened several years ago when rival soup brands Campbell's and Progresso ran ads attacking each other over the controversial flavor enhancer MSG. Campbell's fired the first salvo with ads pointing out that Progresso's "light" soups, unlike Campbell's, contained MSG. Progresso struck back with full-page ads charging that Campbell's had 95 other soups on the market that were made with MSG.

What made this soup squabble especially strange is that Campbell's insists that MSG is perfectly safe. But as the company is well aware, some consumers believe the substance is a poison that causes everything from headaches to autism. Trying to have its MSG and eat it too, Campbell's was in essence saying "shame on Progresso for using the stuff," while adding that line made famous by *Seinfeld*, "not that there's anything wrong with that."

MSG, which stands for "monosodium glutamate," consists of sodium and glutamic acid (aka glutamate), an amino acid that occurs naturally in a wide array of foods, including tomatoes, chicken, Parmesan cheese, and soy sauce. Produced commercially through the fermentation of molasses and sugar beets, MSG is added to soups and other packaged foods to enhance flavor.

MSG first gained public attention in 1968, when a doctor wrote a letter to the *New England Journal of Medicine* complaining of numbness, weakness, and heart palpitations after eating Chinese food. Although he simply listed MSG as one of several possible causes of his mysterious condition, which the journal dubbed "Chinese restaurant syndrome," the damage to MSG's reputation was done.

Over the years, the list of purported effects of MSG has grown to include asthma attacks, migraines, attention deficit disorder, Alzheimer's disease, cancer, and obesity. However, the evidence cited to support such assertions typically comes from animal research, anecdotal reports, and preliminary human studies that have often been contradicted by more rigorous ones. In short, we have little solid proof that MSG causes harm.

Nevertheless, a small percentage of people may be sensitive to MSG. A panel of experts, reviewing the evidence for the FDA, concluded that some individuals might experience temporary symptoms such as headaches, chest pain, numbness, and tingling within an hour of ingesting large amounts of MSG on an empty stomach.

If you're trying to avoid MSG, keep in mind that it can go by other names. Ingredients such as vegetable protein extract and hydrolyzed soy protein, which are found in many packaged foods, contain glutamate. As a result, foods that claim to be free of MSG may actually contain it.

In fact, if you used a magnifying glass to read the fine print of some of those Campbell's ads and packages boasting "no MSG," you could also see this disclaimer: "except for the small amount naturally occurring in yeast extract." Not that there's anything wrong with that.

The taste often used to describe MSG is *umami*, a Japanese term that refers to the savory, satisfying flavor in foods such as steak, mushrooms, and Parmesan cheese. Umami is sometimes called the fifth taste, after sweet, salty, sour, and bitter.

CINNAMON IS EFFECTIVE AGAINST DIABETES

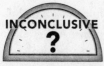 Throughout history, cinnamon has been the subject of many spicy stories, some of them more accurate than others. There's the one, for example, about the Roman emperor Nero, who ordered the burning of a year's supply of cinnamon to express grief over his wife's death—after he killed her. (True.)

And the one about birds from Arabia, known as cinnamon birds because they used cinnamon to build nests. People seeking the highly prized spice lured the birds with big pieces of meat, which the birds took back to their nests. The weight of the meat caused the nests, along with the cinnamon, to fall to the ground. (Not true.)

Then there's the story about the government scientist who fed apple pie to people with diabetes and discovered, much to his surprise, that it lowered their blood sugar levels. The magic ingredient, he figured out, wasn't apples but cinnamon. The part about the pie is true, but whether cinnamon can really help control diabetes remains an open question.

That scientist, Richard Anderson, found that a constituent in cinnamon, known as methylhydroxy chalcone polymer (MHCP), has an insulin-like effect on cells in test tubes. He and his colleagues followed up with a study on 60 subjects who had type 2 diabetes, randomly assigning half to receive one, three, or six grams of cinnamon a day. The other half got dummy pills. After 40 days, the researchers found that the subjects taking cinnamon—at all doses—had lower glucose and cholesterol levels. There were no such changes among the controls.

Since then, other small studies have put cinnamon to the test, and the results have been inconsistent. One possible reason is that different studies have involved different populations: Anderson's research focused on Pakistanis who had poorly controlled diabetes, while other studies were on Europeans and Americans who in some cases didn't have the condition.

What's more, studies have varied in length, and not all have taken into account subjects' diets, which can affect glucose levels. Some scientists suspect that if cinnamon does work, it may be in people with diabetes whose blood sugar levels aren't well controlled.

So far, studies haven't detected any safety problems, though one potential concern is that cinnamon contains coumarin, a compound that in high doses can interfere with blood clotting and harm the kidneys and liver.

If you want to try cinnamon for health reasons, you need at least about a half teaspoon per day; sprinkling a little on your food now and then won't do the trick. Nor, I'm sorry to say, will eating cinnamon rolls. But according to some research, getting a whiff of cinnamon could improve your attention and memory.

That means I now have an excuse to visit Cinnabon stores: The enticing aroma may benefit my health. While I can't verify it, it makes for a great cinnamon story.

There are two main types of cinnamon sold commercially. Ceylon cinnamon, sometimes called "true" cinnamon, has a lighter flavor and is more expensive. Cassia cinnamon, the kind used most often in the United States, has a spicier taste. It's also the type used in most research on blood sugar.

Chapter 5

Down the Garden Path

PRODUCE GROWN LOCALLY IS MOST HEALTHFUL

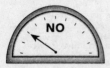 You know a word is hot when it beats out both *upcycling* (the transformation of waste materials into something useful) and *cougar* (an older woman who pursues younger men) for Word of the Year. Yes, there's really such an award, and in 2007 the *New Oxford American Dictionary* bestowed it on *locavore*, meaning someone who buys food grown only within a 100-mile radius of home.

In the last few years, the local food movement has become wildly popular, with everyone from the White House to Walmart jumping on the bandwagon. Enthusiasts are often motivated by the belief that consuming local produce uses less energy and helps protect the planet—a debatable notion that I'll leave to others to address. My focus is the locavores' claim that fruits and veggies from down the road are more healthful than those from across the country or the globe. As one website puts it, "because locally grown produce is freshest, it is more nutritionally complete." To borrow the Sarah Palin–inspired Word of the Year for 2010, I refudiate that.

The nutritional content of produce is determined by a number of factors, including temperature, light, and soil. Though storage and transportation cause some types of produce to lose nutrients, studies show that antioxidant levels may actually *increase* in other cases. As counterintuitive as it seems, this means imported blueberries at your supermarket could have slightly higher nutrient levels than berries right off the bush at your local farmers' market.

Locavores also claim that local produce is more healthful because it's organic. There are two problems with this argument. First, just because produce is grown locally doesn't necessarily mean it's organic. Second, even if it is organic, there's no conclusive evidence that this makes it safer or more nutritious than conventional produce (see "Organic Produce Is More Healthful Than Conventional Produce" on page 71).

Unless you live in Florida or California, being a locavore can make it tough to follow health experts' advice to eat a wide variety of fruits and vegetables, especially in winter. Depending on where you are, nutrient-packed foods like strawberries, bananas, and oranges could be out of reach.

On the other hand, buying local may expand your horticultural horizons by introducing you to fruits and vegetables that aren't commonly sold in supermarkets. It also gives you the chance to learn about where and how the food is grown. But you may have to dig for truthful information. An investigation by a TV station in

Los Angeles revealed widespread fraud at farmers' markets, with some sellers falsely claiming to have grown the food themselves or hawking supposedly organic produce that was actually covered with pesticides.

Of course, most local farmers are honest, and I'm all for supporting them. That's a much better reason for buying local than the food's alleged nutritional superiority. Another is the taste. There's nothing like the flavor of a fresh-picked peach or tomato. My reaction is best expressed by one of the runners-up for the 2010 Word of the Year: *nom nom*, defined as "an expression of delight while eating." Its origin: the sounds made by *Sesame Street*'s Cookie Monster.

Frozen fruits and vegetables are just as nutritious as fresh produce—and perhaps more so, depending on when they were picked and how they were stored. But watch out for sauces and salty seasonings added to some frozen vegetables, which can make them less healthful.

CHOCOLATE IS GOOD FOR YOU

For me, Valentine's Day always feels a little like the movie *Groundhog Day*. Year after year, I seem to encounter the same exact thing: news reports and press releases announcing that it's okay to indulge in chocolate. This once guilty pleasure, we're repeatedly told, has officially reached "superfood" status alongside broccoli, blueberries, and salmon.

Now no one enjoys chocolate more than I do, so you'd think I would welcome the annual lovefest. But the sweet nothings I hear about chocolate's benefits often lack the necessary caveats. As a plant-based food (hence its inclusion in this chapter), chocolate does have potential health benefits. Whether those benefits are real, though, depends on how it's processed and how much you consume.

Cocoa, a main ingredient in chocolate, is made from beans of the cacao plant. Raw cocoa is high in antioxidants known as flavanols, which are also found in red wine, tea, and certain fruits (see "Red Wine Is the Most Beneficial Type of Alcohol" on page 3). Though the evidence overall is mixed, some cohort studies have linked high flavanol intake with lower rates of heart-related deaths.

Processing techniques such as fermentation and roasting, which help improve cocoa's bitter taste, can substantially decrease flavanol levels. Generally, dark chocolate is higher than milk chocolate in flavanols.

Small, short-term experiments—many of them funded by the chocolate industry—show that chocolate (especially the dark variety) can lower blood pressure, improve blood vessel function, reduce inflammation in arteries, and make blood less likely to clot. Even though it's relatively high in saturated fat, studies show chocolate doesn't raise LDL (bad) cholesterol and may even lower it. One reason may be that some of the fat is a type known as stearic acid, which doesn't adversely affect cholesterol levels (see "Saturated Fat Is Bad for Your Heart" on page 29).

What matters most is whether eating chocolate leads to long-term health benefits. And several European cohort studies suggest it may. Research conducted in elderly men, middle-aged adults, and heart attack survivors has linked greater chocolate and cocoa intake to lower rates of heart attacks, strokes, and premature death. But since the chocolate consumed in Europe tends to contain relatively high levels of cocoa, it's unclear whether the findings apply to American chocolate eaters.

In those cohort studies, less than 1 ounce a day was associated with benefits, but many trials have used 3.5 ounces. To get that amount, you'd need to eat two or more standard-size candy bars every day, which add up to 500 additional calories and lots of extra pounds. That's hardly a formula for better health.

If you're eating chocolate for your health, go for the dark kind and make sure that cocoa or chocolate liquor—and not sugar—is the first ingredient listed. Even then, don't expect miracles. Chocolate is, after all, candy—not medicine.

Maybe a better holiday analogy than Groundhog Day is Christmas. If you think about it, Christmas and chocolate have a lot in common: In theory, both can have positive effects on us, but neither fully lives up to all the hype surrounding it. There is one difference, however: We don't get to hear continuous music about chocolate every year.

Despite its reputation as a cause of acne (which is generally undeserved), chocolate may actually be good for your skin. Studies have found that consuming cocoa with very high flavanol levels may protect against damage from the sun's ultraviolet rays, perhaps by increasing blood flow to the skin. Still, chocolate is no substitute for sunscreen and other sun-protection measures.

GARLIC LOWERS CHOLESTEROL

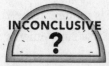

If you're a pitchman for a product known as "stinking rose"—the nickname for garlic—sooner or later you're likely to wind up with a similar label. That's what happened to Larry King, whose radio ads for Garlique-brand garlic pills earned him the appellation "garlic breath" among online posters. It didn't help that Donald Trump said to King during an interview, "Do you mind if I sit back a little bit because your breath is very bad. It really is."

In those ads for Garlique, King claimed that garlic "has been clinically shown to maintain healthy cholesterol levels"—a euphemism for *lowers cholesterol*. By using such language, the manufacturer avoided having to provide evidence to the FDA. A wise move, since the claims don't quite pass the smell test.

Animal research suggests that garlic may work by inhibiting the body's production of cholesterol or decreasing its absorption in the intestines. But human studies have produced inconsistent findings. In a review of 10 randomized trials, 6 of them showed garlic to be effective, reducing total and LDL (bad) cholesterol by about 10 percent. A 2001 meta-analysis of studies found that garlic slightly lowered cholesterol for three months but didn't appear to work when taken for six months. A more recent meta-analysis, this one of 13 trials, concluded that garlic has little or no benefit.

One possible reason for the inconsistencies is that some studies have put restrictions on subjects' diets, while others have not. Because diet can affect cholesterol levels, the failure to control this variable can skew research results.

Another explanation is that studies have involved different types of garlic supplements, some of which may be more effective than others. The active ingredient in fresh garlic is thought to be a compound known as allicin, and tests have found that supplements vary widely in the amounts they provide.

To get more definitive answers, investigators conducted a head-to-head comparison. Nearly 200 subjects were randomly assigned to get raw garlic (blended with a spread on sandwiches), one of two types of supplements, or placebos. All subjects had moderately elevated LDL levels.

After six months, people taking garlic, in whatever form, were no better off than those getting placebos. And there were unpleasant side effects: About 8 percent of subjects who took supplements reported experiencing gas "often," and 57 percent in the raw garlic group complained of bad breath and body odor "almost always."

That's a pretty high price to pay for something that may or may not be effective. As for Larry King's breath, Donald Trump claims that he really didn't mean what he said about it. Nevertheless, King's garlic breath rap lives on, a side effect of those radio ads. I hope the paycheck was worth the price.

While cholesterol lowering is perhaps garlic's most publicized health effect, there's also some evidence that it can reduce blood pressure and prevent blood clots and colds.

RAW VEGGIES ARE MORE NUTRITIOUS THAN COOKED

 Medical journals are about the last place most of us would go for entertaining reading. But if you look closely enough, you can find some pretty bizarre stories—medical versions of News of the Weird. And sometimes these odd tales reveal truths far more compellingly than any study could.

Take the case of the 88-year-old woman who showed up at the emergency room near death due to an overdose of . . . raw vegetables. In an account published in the *New England Journal of Medicine*, doctors noted that she was extremely lethargic and unable to walk or swallow. She was diagnosed with myxedema coma, a life-threatening condition caused by very low thyroid function, and admitted to intensive care.

It turns out she had been eating huge amounts of uncooked bok choy—a type of cabbage—in hopes of controlling her diabetes. The vegetable contains compounds called glucosinolates that when broken down by the body can adversely affect the thyroid gland. Hence the woman's problem. She could likely have avoided it if she'd cooked her bok choy, because cooking prevents these compounds from breaking down.

As the story illustrates, raw vegetables aren't always better for you, and in some cases cooking may make them more healthful. In addition to increasing digestibility, it can boost levels of certain nutrients. Whether a particular vegetable is more nutritious cooked or raw depends on the vegetable, the nutrient, and the cooking method.

For example, research shows we get more of the antioxidant lycopene (which has been linked to a lower risk of prostate cancer and heart disease) from cooked tomatoes than from raw ones (see "Tomatoes Prevent Prostate Cancer" on page 77). Heat breaks down tomatoes' cell walls, which releases more lycopene and helps the body better absorb it. Likewise, cooking carrots, green beans, celery, spinach, peppers, and other veggies can increase levels of certain antioxidants.

On the other hand, cooking can destroy vitamin C. How much is lost varies according to the cooking method. One study, comparing different ways of cooking broccoli, found that boiling lowered vitamin C levels by about a third. Microwaving and pressure-cooking, in contrast, retained virtually all of the vitamin.

Microwaving also beat boiling in a study that analyzed the effects of different cooking methods on antioxidant levels in 20 vegetables. It's notable that the researchers didn't use water during microwaving; a previous study that did add water found that antioxidants leached out of broccoli into the water. Steaming can be a good option too as long as you don't cook too long.

If you enjoy chomping on crudités, have at it. But you don't need to eat like Bugs Bunny all the time to get the benefits of veggies. The best approach is to consume a wide variety in whatever form you most enjoy. That way, you'll eat more.

Luckily, the elderly woman who OD'd on vegetables recovered. She was released to a nursing home, where they presumably limited her intake of raw bok choy. If the food there was anything like that at most other healthcare facilities, there was no such limit on mushy, overcooked vegetables.

Eating vegetables along with fat, such as oil in salad dressing, can help the body better absorb the veggies' nutrients.

ORGANIC PRODUCE IS MORE HEALTHFUL THAN CONVENTIONAL PRODUCE

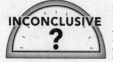

Not long ago, if you wanted to buy organic foods, you'd have to go to a farmers' market or a hole-in-the-wall health-food store run by an ex-hippie. Today, you can find organic food in virtually every supermarket, and even in convenience stores whose main offerings include beer, Cheez-Its, and Ho Hos.

Though organic items can cost two or three times as much as regular foods, nearly 40 percent of Americans say they buy organic at least occasionally according to one survey. Why? The same survey shows that more than 90 percent of the most loyal buyers believe organic food is better for the environment. And virtually 100 percent think it's better for their health.

On the first point, they're correct. Organic farming, which shuns conventional pesticides and petroleum-based fertilizers, results in less soil depletion and pollution than conventional methods. That's a subject for another book, however. When it comes to health, I'm sorry to have to burst the believers' (ozone-free) bubble, but science isn't entirely on their side.

Here's what we know: Organic produce has fewer chemical residues than the conventional kind (though levels aren't necessarily zero). At a gut level, this seems like a good thing. The idea that your blueberries contain a helping of bug poison can be unsettling, to say the least.

In larger amounts, chemicals used in conventional agriculture have been shown to cause acute poisoning and other adverse effects in people—an issue of special relevance to farm workers and their offspring. But there's far less clarity regarding the traces of chemicals to which consumers are routinely exposed through food. While some preliminary studies provide hints that low levels might lead to neurological or behavioral problems in children, there's no hard proof for this.

The science is similarly uncertain regarding the alleged nutritional superiority of organic produce. Proponents claim that organic farming methods result in higher levels of antioxidants (including vitamin C) and other nutrients. Some research, in fact, supports this assertion. But a review of more than 50 studies found no nutritional advantages for organic. And even if organic fruits and veggies are more nutritious, it's unknown whether the differences are large enough to really matter.

There's greater certainty regarding another popular notion— that organic produce is less prone to contamination from harmful bacteria like *Salmonella* or *E. coli*. It's simply not true. Nor is it correct that packaged foods are necessarily more healthful just because they're organic. Slapping an organic label onto cookies or chips may be a good marketing gimmick, but it doesn't transform them into health foods. They're still junk.

If you like the idea of eating organic but can't stomach the price, consider going organic for produce like apples, strawberries, and peaches, which tend to have the highest levels of pesticides. For those that have low levels, such as onions, avocados, and pineapples, stick with conventional.

That way, you'll have money left over for those healthy organic Ho Hos.

Research shows that an organic label can have a so-called halo effect, positively affecting our perceptions of a food. In one experiment, people who ate cookies, potato chips, and yogurt that were labeled "organic" judged these to be lower in calories and fat, higher in fiber, and more nutritious than the identical items without an organic label.

ACAI BERRIES HELP YOU LOSE WEIGHT

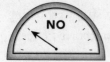 Sasha Conrad is a success story—or so it would seem. On her blog, the working mother of two children tells how acai berries helped her lose 25 pounds, and she's posted photos to prove it. Nadia Johnson achieved similar results, which she also documented with before-and-after pictures on her blog. More than 60 other women have posted similar stories, along with photos, on their blogs as well.

Sounds impressive until you know this: The pictures are all of the same woman. Her photo was purchased from a stock photography library and digitally altered to make her look thin for the "after" pictures. What's more, many of these blogs contain identical wording. It's all a big scam to sell acai berries, which was exposed by a legitimate blog called Wafflesatnoon.com.

As for claims that acai berries promote weight loss, they're no more believable than the bogus blogs.

Acai (pronounced *ah-sigh-EE*) is a berry from Brazil that's been widely touted in the United States for its health-enhancing powers. In addition to removing toxins and increasing energy, the alleged benefits include burning fat, reducing food cravings, and boosting metabolism. Typically the berry is sold in the form of juice (for as much as $40 a bottle), capsules, or powder.

What supposedly makes acai berries so beneficial is their high levels of antioxidants, which help fight harmful free radicals. While some studies show that the berries are rich in antioxidants, other research has found that acai juice ranks in the middle of the antioxidant scale, below Concord grape juice but above apple juice.

Whatever the case, antioxidant activity doesn't tell us whether the berries have benefits. That requires human studies showing that they actually lead to weight loss or other purported effects, and so far such research is lacking.

This hasn't stopped claims on the Internet that acai berries can help you lose 20 pounds in 20 days or that they result in "450 percent more weight loss than dieting and exercising alone." Some sites falsely claim that Oprah Winfrey endorses their products, which has prompted her to file a lawsuit against a number of marketers.

As long as you don't count on it to melt away pounds or perform other health miracles, acai juice is a perfectly fine beverage. Just watch out for brands with added sugar and calories. Also, beware of sites that offer "risk-free" trials for acai products. The

Center for Science in the Public Interest reports that many consumers who signed up for such deals have been hit with monthly charges of $80 or more on their credit cards, which continued after they tried to cancel.

To warn others, maybe these folks should post blogs with pictures of their shrinking wallets. If they're interested, I'd be happy to sell them photos.

Like acai berries, pomegranates are touted as so-called superfoods with a host of health benefits. Though there's more science behind the claims for pomegranates (especially juice), it's still preliminary, and there's no hard evidence that pomegranates or acai berries are any better for you than other berries.

SOY WARDS OFF CANCER

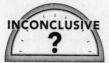

Prisoners, like hospital patients, generally have little good to say about the food they're served. But inmates in Illinois claim their grub is so gross that it amounts to cruel and unusual punishment. The complaint isn't that the mystery meat is cold or that the hash is bland, however. It's about what the food contains: soy.

To cut costs, Illinois prisons are using soy in everything from sausages to sloppy joes. The prisoners have taken their grievance to court, alleging that all this soy is sickening them with a host of ailments.

If you believe one ex-prisoner, however, soy may be saving their lives. Michael Milken, the former junk bond king who spent two years in the slammer, credits soy with putting his prostate cancer in remission. In a cookbook that he coauthored, Milken notes that Americans have a much higher incidence of prostate cancer than men in Asia. Citing the lack of soy in our diet as a main reason, he sticks it in everything from salad dressings to chocolate shakes.

The theory is that substances in soy called isoflavones, which are plant estrogens, can inhibit the development of prostate, breast, and other hormone-related cancers. Some animal research supports this idea when it comes to prostate cancer. But human studies have been mixed. A few cohort studies have found that men consuming more soy have lower rates of prostate cancer, while others have turned up no association.

With breast cancer, the story is even more complicated. A few animal and test-tube studies have shown that soy may actually *promote* the growth of breast tumors. However, there's no hard evidence for this from human studies, some of which suggest that soy may be beneficial. For example, a cohort study of 5,000 breast cancer survivors in China linked high soy intake to a decreased risk of cancer recurrence and death. However, other cohort studies have found no connection between soy and breast cancer.

One possible reason for the inconsistencies in breast and prostate cancer research is that different studies have involved different populations consuming different amounts of soy. Generally, studies in Asian countries, where intake is relatively high, have yielded more favorable results for soy than has research in Western countries.

Another factor may be the type of soy consumed. In Asian

countries, the main sources are typically foods such as tofu, miso (soybean paste), and natto (fermented soybeans), which are made from whole soybeans. In contrast, we in the West get much of our soy from extracts of the bean (often labeled as soy protein isolate) used in processed foods. Some researchers theorize that this form of soy is less beneficial or possibly even harmful.

Timing may play a role as well. Animal studies as well as several case-control studies hint that eating soy early in life may offer more protection against breast cancer than consuming it in adulthood.

While we can't say for sure whether soy prevents cancer, it's a good source of protein and can be part of a healthy diet. Maybe the state of Illinois should enlist Michael Milken to sell the prisoners on soy. If he can do for soy what he did for junk bonds, the inmates will soon be yelling for more.

People with low thyroid levels may want to go easy on soy. Studies suggest that a high soy intake can further impair their thyroid function. Other foods, such as peanuts and raw cruciferous vegetables (broccoli, cabbage, Brussels sprouts), may have a similar effect.

TOMATOES PREVENT PROSTATE CANCER

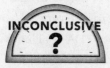

Even if you don't like tomatoes, you have to feel some sympathy for them. Angry mobs use them as projectiles. Moviemakers portray them as vicious killers. Society won't even accept them for what they really are—a fruit, not a vegetable.

Recently, tomatoes have gotten a badly needed morale boost, earning recognition as a so-called superfood largely because of their purported ability to fight prostate cancer. I hate to keep a good man (or food) down, but the accolade may be undeserved.

Tomatoes are relatively high in the antioxidant lycopene, which gives them their red color. Lab research suggests it may protect against cancer, and some studies (though not all) measuring lycopene in blood have found that men with high levels are less prone to prostate cancer.

The strongest evidence for the tomato–prostate connection comes from a Harvard cohort study that followed more than 47,000 male health professionals. It found that those who consumed tomato products (typically tomato sauce) most frequently had a slightly lower risk of prostate cancer. But another large cohort study, funded by the National Cancer Institute, showed no such benefit. The results from other cohort and case-control studies have been mixed.

The FDA, reviewing the evidence in response to a request by the H.J. Heinz Company to put health claims on tomato products, concluded there was a "very low level of comfort" that tomatoes protect against prostate cancer. Nevertheless, the agency gave the green light to a claim that "very limited and preliminary scientific research suggests that eating one-half to one cup of tomatoes and/or tomato sauce a week may reduce the risk of prostate cancer."

Manufacturers are also required to add this: "FDA concludes that there is little scientific evidence supporting this claim." Needless to say, Heinz and other companies aren't exactly jumping to plaster this tangled message on their tomato paste.

So why the scientific confusion? For starters, the size of the benefit—if it exists—appears to be relatively modest, so small studies may not be able to detect it. What's more, the amount of lycopene we get from tomato foods can vary depending on, among other things, whether they're cooked or accompanied by fat. (Both increase the body's ability to absorb lycopene.) Such details aren't always fully captured in food questionnaires that scientists use to measure what people eat.

None of this uncertainty has stopped scientists in Europe and the United States from developing special tomatoes with very high levels of lycopene. Whether there's consumer demand remains to be seen, but at least tomatoes now have their own version of a superhero. Maybe it can save the world in a future *Killer Tomatoes* movie.

Tomatoes aren't the only produce rich in lycopene. One wedge of watermelon (about a sixteenth of a melon) contains more lycopene than four medium-size tomatoes. But to get the most out of your melon, serve it at room temperature. One study found that watermelons sitting at 70°F have up to 40 percent more lycopene than those at 55°F.

Chapter 6

Meaty or Fishy?

RED MEAT IS BAD FOR YOU

Growing up, most of us were subjected to all kinds of lessons from our mothers. Some of these "momisms" were sound (don't cross the street before looking both ways), while others weren't (don't cross your eyes or they'll get stuck that way). Then there were the edicts that fell in between, such as wear clean underwear in case you get into an accident. The advice was sensible, but the rationale was incomplete. (Mom—of all people—forgot a much more important reason: good hygiene.)

The conventional advice about red meat is similarly deficient. We're often told to avoid it because too much is bad for our hearts. Indeed, research does suggest that a high-meat diet poses a health risk—but the most established threat is cancer, not heart disease.

More than a dozen cohort studies have linked a high intake of red meat—defined as beef, pork, lamb, or anything made from them, like hamburgers, sausage, or chili—to an increased risk of colorectal cancer. For example, a European study of 478,000 men and women found that colorectal cancer was more common among those who consumed the most red meat (about 5.5 ounces or more a day) compared to those who ate the least (less than 1 ounce).

Research has also associated meat eating with other types of cancer, including lung, liver, and esophagus, though this evidence is less conclusive than that for colorectal cancer.

One possible culprit behind the meat–cancer connection is the type of iron (known as heme iron) in red meat. During digestion, it contributes to the formation of potentially cancer-causing substances in the gut known as N-nitroso compounds. Other suspects include chemicals known as heterocyclic amines (HCAs), which form when meat is cooked at high temperatures (see "Well-Done Meat Causes Cancer" on page 84).

Scientists suspect that these same factors, along with red meat's relatively high levels of saturated fat (see "Saturated Fat Is Bad for Your Heart" on page 29), may be responsible for any association with heart disease. But overall, the evidence linking red meat to heart disease is mixed. Some studies—including one that followed 84,000 women for 26 years—have found that those who eat more meat are at increased risk of heart disease. But when researchers pooled data from 20 studies involving 1.2 million people, they turned up no association.

These scientists did find that processed meats, which include bacon, ham, sausage, and hot dogs, were associated with a higher risk of both heart disease and diabetes. Other research has linked them to colon cancer as well. (Nitrates and nitrites, which are used to preserve, flavor, and color many processed meats, are suspected culprits.) One large study found that people who ate the most processed—and red—meat were slightly more likely to die prematurely.

None of this means you need to forgo meat completely. A small steak or hamburger once or twice a week is likely fine, as is an occasional hot dog. Just remember Mom's lesson about everything in moderation. It's hard to argue with that one.

Pork, which was once billed "the Other White Meat" in industry ads, can in fact be as lean as poultry—but only if you choose the right cut. A four-ounce piece of pork tenderloin (with the fat trimmed) has about the same amount of saturated fat and calories as a chicken breast with skin. But a four-ounce pork chop has more than twice the fat and nearly 50 percent more calories, making it comparable to sirloin steak.

GRASS-FED BEEF IS MORE HEALTHFUL THAN GRAIN-FED BEEF

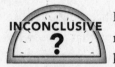

During piano lessons as a kid, I was taught the mnemonic "Every Good Boy Does Fine" for the lines in the treble clef. Back then I had no idea what this expression meant, and I still don't. The one for spaces in the bass clef—"All Cows Eat Grass"—made far more sense. But as a lesson about cattle farming, it was a bit off key.

Cows in the United States are raised mainly on corn and other grains, not grass. In recent years, though, grass-fed beef has become increasingly popular, in part because it's touted as being more healthful than the conventional kind. While grass-fed beef appears to have some nutritional advantages, it's unclear whether the higher price buys you better health.

As ruminants, cows are designed to live on grass. That's what they're fed early in life, but as they get older, they're usually sent to feedlots and put on a grain diet to fatten them up as quickly as possible. The result is that beef from grain-fed cattle is higher in fat overall—and, consequently, more tender (and some would say tastier)—than that from cattle eating only grass their entire lives.

Both grass- and grain-fed beef contain saturated fat, the type that's often associated with a greater risk of heart disease (see "Saturated Fat Is Bad for Your Heart" on page 29). But in grass-fed beef, a higher percentage of the saturated fat is a type known as stearic acid, which does not raise cholesterol levels.

In addition, grass-fed beef is richer in omega-3 fatty acids than conventional beef, and research shows that subjects who consume grass-fed beef have higher blood levels of this good fat than those who eat conventional beef. Still, the amount of omega-3s in beef pales in comparison to that in fish such as salmon. What's more, this fat comes in a form known as alpha-linolenic acid (ALA), whose benefits aren't as well documented as those of the omega-3s in fish (see "Fish Oil Prevents Heart Disease" on page 23).

Grass-fed beef also has an edge when it comes to a type of fat called conjugated linoleic acid (CLA), which is often claimed to prevent heart disease, cancer, diabetes, and obesity. However, most of the evidence comes from lab and animal studies, so it's hard to draw any firm conclusions about its effects on human health.

As for safety, we often hear that conventional beef is more likely than grass-fed beef to cause foodborne illness. That's because grain makes the stomachs of cattle more acidic, and the acidic environment is thought to lead to a higher prevalence of harmful *E. coli* bacteria. While some studies have found this to be true, others suggest that grass-fed beef is just as likely to be contaminated as the conventional kind.

One thing we know for certain is that cattle fed an all-grass diet rarely require antibiotics, while those raised on grain routinely get the drugs. Many scientists believe that the widespread use of antibiotics in animals is contributing to the rise of drug-resistant bacteria, so choosing grass-fed over grain-fed beef may be one small way of promoting better public health.

Instead of the "All Cows Eat Grass" mnemonic, maybe it should be "Antibiotic-Fed Cows Eat Grain." It's certainly more accurate. I'm just not sure it would go over so well with second-graders.

Beef labeled "organic" isn't necessarily grass-fed. The term *organic* means the cows don't receive antibiotics or hormones and eat only organic feed. But that feed can be grain or grass.

WELL-DONE MEAT CAUSES CANCER

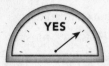 You've probably heard of the Iron Chef, the French Chef, and the Naked Chef. Call me the Nervous Chef. While I enjoy having friends over for cookouts, I worry that I'll undercook the meat and send

them off with *Salmonella* as a party favor. As a result, I typically end up grilling (and grilling) until everything is well done. I may not be doing my friends any favors, however. Charred chicken or burgers, while eliminating one health risk, may pose another: cancer.

Cooking food at high temperatures or until it's well done can produce chemicals called heterocyclic amines (HCAs), which cause cancer in lab animals. HCAs form in meats—including beef, pork, poultry, and, to a lesser extent, seafood—but not veggies or tofu. Longer cooking times result in more HCAs. So do higher temperatures, which is why grilling, barbecuing, and broiling tend to produce the highest levels of HCAs. Low-temperature cooking methods, such as stewing and poaching, result in virtually none of the chemicals.

A number of population and case-control studies have looked at the effects of HCAs on human health. Some have found no association, but most have linked high intakes of well-done meat to various types of cancer, including colorectal, breast, prostate, pancreatic, lung, and stomach.

Further evidence comes from several large cohort studies. In one, for example, men who consumed at least a third of an ounce a day of well-done meat had a slightly higher risk of prostate cancer than men who ate none. Another, known as the NIH-AARP Diet and Health Study, found a small increase in the risk of pancreatic cancer among men who ate the most grilled and barbecued red meat. There was no association with meat that was sautéed, baked, or microwaved.

Overall, the evidence is strong enough to warrant taking precautions. Marinating meat before slapping it on the grill can reduce the formation of HCAs, as can zapping it in the microwave for a minute or two before cooking. Don't use pan drippings for gravy or basting because they can have high levels of HCAs.

When you grill, keep the heat down, avoid flame flare-ups, flip the food frequently, and remove it before it's well done or charred. To make sure your food is sufficiently cooked—my big concern— use a thermometer.

Come to think of it, I've never used that digital meat thermometer sitting in my kitchen drawer. It's time to start. Maybe the friend who gave it to me was trying to tell me something.

Because they're cooked quickly, fast-food burgers and chicken tend to be low in HCAs.

KOSHER MEAT IS MORE WHOLESOME THAN CONVENTIONAL MEAT

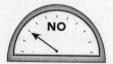 When Benjamin Franklin uttered the aphorism "out of adversity comes opportunity," it's safe to assume he didn't have kosher food in mind. But he might as well have.

Sales of kosher food have soared in recent years thanks to fears about food contamination. In a survey by Mintel, a market research firm, consumers named "safety" along with "quality" and "general healthfulness" as the main motives for buying kosher. A mere 14 percent of respondents cited religious reasons, an indication that kosher's biggest customers may now be those who don't know a knish from gefilte fish.

Under Jewish dietary law, animals are slaughtered by having their throats slit, a process that's claimed to result in a quicker, more humane death. Because cattle aren't first stunned with a bolt to the head, as is typically done in conventional slaughtering, there's less risk of brains scattering to other parts of the carcass. In theory, this means a lower risk of the human form of mad cow disease, which is caused by proteins from infected brain tissue. However, the disease is relatively rare—there have been only a few hundred cases reported worldwide—so the advantages of kosher in this regard are fairly minimal.

Kosher rules also require blood to be removed from meat through salting and rinsing. One study found that this process reduces levels of *Salmonella* in poultry, but other research has found *Listeria*, another type of bacteria, to be *more* prevalent in kosher chicken than in the conventional kind. While the benefits of salting on health are unclear, there is a definite downside: higher sodium levels, which may pose a problem for those prone to high blood pressure.

Kosher food producers claim to answer to a "higher authority," as the Hebrew National slogan puts it. In some cases, this means their meat contains no hormones, antibiotics, or artificial ingredients. But none of this is required by Jewish law. Kosher certification does not govern what type of feed animals receive, nor does it mandate how much space, sunshine, or exercise they get.

As a result, *kosher* isn't necessarily synonymous with *organic*. Nor does it guarantee that the food is any safer, purer, or better for you than the conventional kind. Next time you hear such a claim, it would be wise to remember another of Ben Franklin's sayings:

"Believe none of what you hear and half of what you see." Unless, of course, it comes directly from that higher authority.

The label "free range" on poultry means only that the animals have access to the outdoors. There's no guarantee that they actually go outside or spend significant amounts of time there. Like the term *kosher, free range* doesn't necessarily ensure that the animals are treated more humanely or that the meat is less prone to contamination.

FARMED SALMON IS LESS HEALTHFUL THAN WILD-CAUGHT SALMON

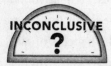 For some people, supermarket shopping is enjoyable. For me, it's mentally draining because it always sparks a fight inside my head. In one corner is my health-conscious self, which says I should buy whatever is most healthful. In the other is my cost-conscious self, which balks at spending a dime more than I have to.

This drama frequently plays out as I ponder the salmon selections. The dialogue (which, luckily for the person behind the counter, is silent) goes something like this:

VOICE 1: Buy the wild salmon instead of the farm raised. So what if it's twice as expensive? Your health is worth it.

VOICE 2: He's crazy. Farmed is perfectly fine. Save your money.

VOICE 1: Is saving a few bucks really worth the greater risk
 of cancer that comes from contaminated farmed fish?
VOICE 2: You're a sucker if you fall for that.

Once the noise subsides, here's what my rational self has to say: Research shows that overall, farmed salmon is more likely to be contaminated than the wild kind. A large study published in the journal *Science* found that farmed salmon contained higher levels of dioxins, pesticides, and industrial chemicals known as PCBs. Amounts varied according to the fish's origin: The worst offenders came from Scotland and the Faroe Islands, while the least contaminated farmed samples were from Chile and Washington State.

The source of the pollutants is the farmed fish's chow. When small fish are ground up to make fishmeal, as is often done, any chemicals they contain become more concentrated. The same is true when oil is extracted from fish and used as food.

PCBs and other pollutants have been shown to cause cancer in animals, and some studies suggest that workers exposed to high levels of the chemicals may be more prone to cancer. Based on federal safety standards and their own findings, the researchers who conducted that study in *Science* estimated that eating farmed salmon more than once a month or so poses an increased cancer risk. But there's no evidence directly linking farmed fish consumption to cancer.

Further muddying the waters is the fact that contamination levels may be declining as more farms switch to other types of fish food. What's more, fish isn't our primary source of PCBs and dioxins; we typically get more from meat, dairy products, and vegetables.

One advantage of farmed salmon is that it contains higher levels of heart-healthy omega-3 fatty acids than does wild salmon (see "Fish Oil Prevents Heart Disease" on page 23). And some research shows that farmed salmon may have less mercury than the wild kind, though both are relatively low in mercury (see "Mercury in Sushi Is Toxic" below).

On the other hand, wild salmon may be better for the environment, since salmon farming can spread waste and disease into the ocean. That's why when I buy farmed salmon, I try to get it from places that require suppliers to meet strict environmental standards. I also grill the seller about where the fish came from. (Atlantic salmon is always farmed, Alaskan salmon is always wild, and Pacific salmon can be either.)

Gathering such information can make my decision about what to buy a little easier. Then it's time to seek out those free samples of cookies, cheese, or bread that the store hands out. After putting up with those annoying voices, I figure I'm entitled.

Cooking salmon, trimming the fat, and removing the skin can reduce contaminant levels by up to half.

MERCURY IN SUSHI IS TOXIC

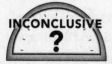

The actor Jeremy Piven is best known for playing Ari Gold, the explosive agent on the HBO series *Entourage*. If Piven ever wondered what it's like to be the recipient of Ari's venomous attacks, he found out when he quit a Broadway show in 2008 because of alleged mercury poisoning from sushi.

Many people, including the show's producers, were highly skeptical, if not downright derisive. A *Daily Beast* headline mockingly referred to Piven's "fishy excuse," while the *New York Post* declared, "Piven's Fish Tale Begins to Stink." Though some speculated that Piven's reported symptoms of nausea, dizziness, and weakness were due more to his love of partying than to fish, the episode heightened concerns among sushi eaters that their beloved tako and toro could be toxic.

Mercury, which is released into the atmosphere by industrial plants, falls into water, where microbes convert it to a form known as methylmercury. Fish then absorb it while feeding. Large fish with long life spans tend to have the highest mercury levels.

When the *New York Times* tested local sushi samples in 2008, it found that 25 percent of the surveyed stores and restaurants sold tuna with mercury levels exceeding the FDA's "action level"—the point at which the agency can act to remove food from the market. Tests of sushi from other cities have yielded similar results.

As alarming as this sounds, it's not clear whether such levels actually pose a health risk. We know from studies of mercury poisonings in Japan and Iraq that prenatal exposure to extremely high mercury levels can cause neurological damage in children. In places like the Faroe Islands and the Seychelles Islands, where people eat large amounts of fish and are typically exposed to mercury levels about 10 times higher than those among U.S. residents, research findings have been inconsistent.

Some of these studies have linked prenatal exposure to lower scores on children's brain development tests, but others have turned up no association. Research in the United States and Great Britain has found that the kids whose mothers consumed more fish scored *higher* on cognitive tests, suggesting that the benefits of fish may outweigh any harms from the mercury it contains.

To be on the safe side, the FDA advises women who are pregnant, are nursing, or may become pregnant to eat up to two fish meals a week but to avoid high-mercury fish—shark, swordfish, king mackerel, and tilefish—and to limit their intake of albacore tuna to six ounces per week. The advisory applies to young children as well.

For everyone else, fishing for answers is harder. A few population and case-control studies in adults have linked lower-level mercury exposure to subtle neurological deficits; other research has found no such effects. Likewise, research is conflicting as to whether mercury in fish is associated with a higher risk of heart disease. We do have relatively strong and consistent evidence, however, that fish itself is *good* for your heart (see "Fish Oil Prevents Heart Disease" on page 23).

The moral of this muddle is to keep eating sushi if you enjoy it. To hedge your bets, watch your intake of tuna and instead choose fish that's lower in mercury, like salmon. That way, there's no chance you'll wind up like Jeremy Piven and have to quit your job because of sushi sickness. Then again, maybe it's just the excuse you've been looking for.

Canned white tuna has about three times more mercury than chunk light. That's because the species used for white tuna, albacore, is larger and accumulates more mercury than skipjack, which is used for chunk light. Canned salmon has less mercury than both types of tuna.

Chapter 7

Milking the Science

YOGURT IMPROVES DIGESTION

 Judging from the long lines, you'd think that the frozen yogurt joint near my house is handing out cash. Since the yogurt's taste isn't anything special, I suspect what attracts many in my earthy-crunchy neighborhood is the store's promotion of its product as a health food, with signs screaming "Live Culture!" Sometimes I wonder whether any puzzled patrons see this and think an opera performance is about to start.

In fact, it means the yogurt supposedly contains billions of "good" bacteria, known as probiotics, that fight harmful ones and help us digest food. Thanks to Jamie Lee Curtis's ads for Activia yogurt (or perhaps *Saturday Night Live*'s widely viewed parodies of them), one of the most familiar claims for yogurt with probiotics is that it can help alleviate digestive problems. Whether that's true depends on which probiotics and which digestive problems you're talking about.

We have good evidence from clinical trials that certain types of probiotics—including LGG bacteria and *L. reuteri*—are effective against acute diarrhea in children. Solid research also shows that LGG and *S. boulardii* can prevent or ease diarrhea due to antibiotic use.

There's decent—though less conclusive—evidence that certain probiotics (including one called VSL#3) may improve symptoms such as bloating and gas in people with irritable bowel syndrome. Likewise, some (though not all) research suggests that taking probiotics may prevent travelers' diarrhea, the kind you get from contaminated food or water in a foreign country.

When it comes to constipation—or "irregularity," as Jamie Lee Curtis euphemistically refers to it in those ads—the case is far less compelling. Studies funded by Activia's manufacturer, Dannon, show that three daily servings of the product decrease "transit time." While this sounds as though eating yogurt can shorten your commute to work (wouldn't that be nice?), what it really means is that food moves more quickly through the digestive tract. However, this isn't necessarily the same as reducing occasional constipation.

A review of the research on probiotics and constipation found that the evidence overall is limited, and that any benefits may be minimal. For example, in one study, taking probiotics resulted in a grand total of one more stool per week. Not exactly a royal flush.

Vague claims on yogurt labels, such as "regulates digestive health," are best ignored. Such language—which avoids saying explicitly that yogurt can treat or prevent a condition—allows companies to claim that a product has health benefits without having to provide any proof to the FDA.

By themselves, the terms *probiotic* and *live, active cultures* don't tell you whether a yogurt can help with your particular issue. Look for the full scientific names of the probiotics as well as the seal of the National Yogurt Association, which indicates that the doses are sufficiently large.

My local frozen yogurt shop doesn't disclose any of this, but they do have signs saying their product is "healthy." Evidently, that—or the granola toppings—are enough to keep the customers coming back.

Greek yogurt, which is strained and therefore thicker than regular yogurt, has more than twice as much protein. But it's also a bit higher in calories and lower in calcium.

RAW MILK IS BETTER FOR YOU THAN PASTEURIZED MILK

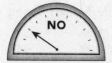

We humans can have some curious priorities when it comes to our health and safety. For example, some of us worry about being attacked by sharks at the beach (a minuscule risk) while blithely basking in the sun all day and exposing ourselves to skin cancer. Others fret over getting brain tumors from cell phones (an unproven peril) but think nothing of talking and texting while driving.

And then there's drinking unpasteurized (also known as raw)

milk. Some raw milk enthusiasts, shunning pasteurized milk because they say it's unhealthful, extol the alleged health benefits of raw milk—everything from preventing allergies to treating cancer—while disregarding its potentially life-threatening dangers.

Pasteurization involves heating milk to high temperatures to kill bacteria. Before the process was widely adopted, contaminated milk routinely made people sick. Today, milk-related disease outbreaks are rare. While other advances—such as healthier animals, improved farm sanitation, and better refrigeration methods—have also enhanced milk safety, they aren't foolproof. For example, a little cow poop can still sometimes get mixed in during milking (sorry if you're reading this while eating your cereal), so pasteurization is an important backstop.

Because the process kills beneficial bacteria along with the harmful kind, raw milk proponents claim that pasteurization makes the beverage less healthful or even harmful. They also say it strips milk of health-enhancing enzymes, vitamins, and minerals, though analyses show nutrient levels to be about the same in raw and pasteurized milk.

Several studies among European farm children have found that those who drink raw milk are less likely to have allergies, asthma, and eczema. However, these are population studies, which show only statistical associations and may miss other aspects of farm life that are actually responsible.

There's even less evidence for other purported benefits, which include the prevention or treatment of autism, tooth decay, behavioral problems, digestive disorders, cancer, and heart disease. As "proof," raw milk advocates typically cite testimonials by milk drinkers and tales of healers from centuries past who used milk as a cure-all. Not exactly rock-solid science.

We do have hard data about the hazards of raw milk, however. From 1998 to 2008, there were two reported deaths and more than 1,600 illnesses in the United States due to raw milk or raw milk products contaminated with bacteria such as *Campylobacter*, *Salmonella*, and *E. coli*. In many cases, the victims—often young children—had to be hospitalized, sometimes with kidney failure.

As raw milk proponents are quick to point out, there have been reports of illness from pasteurized milk as well. But raw milk clearly poses a much greater risk. It accounts for 70 percent or more of dairy-related disease outbreaks in the United States but less than 3 percent of the milk sold.

Whatever the possible health advantages of raw milk, it hardly seems worth the risk. Now if you'll excuse me, I need to go hang gliding. I hear it's an excellent way to lower your cholesterol.

Though goats produce less manure than cows, raw milk from goats isn't necessarily any safer than that from cows. Contaminated raw goat's milk has caused outbreaks that involved serious illness, especially in children.

SOY MILK IS MORE HEALTHFUL THAN COW'S MILK

If you'd asked me 20 years ago what I thought of soy milk, my answer would have included words like *weird*, *disgusting*, and *undrinkable*. In reality, I had no idea what it tasted like because I'd never tried it. But I knew that it had a brownish tinge and was sold in strange boxes not too far from the kelp and wheat germ in health-food stores. That was enough to tell me I wanted no part of it.

Today, I pour it on my cereal every morning. So what prompted the change? An extreme milk makeover. Packaging the beverage in chilled milk cartons and selling it in supermarket dairy cases, the makers of Silk turned soy milk into something that seemed more normal.

As a result, I was willing to try it, and like Mikey in the old Life cereal commercials, I liked it. Plenty of other people apparently had the same experience. Since its image overhaul in 1996, soy milk has become a cash cow. Fueling sales is the perception that it's more healthful than regular milk. Whether that's true, though, depends on what yardstick you use.

Let's start with calories: You get about 100 in a cup of plain soy milk from a carton, roughly the same number in skim milk. Make that whole milk, however, and soy is the better choice. As for fat, soy has an edge here as well: Unlike skim milk, it contains unsaturated fat that's thought to be beneficial. And unlike whole milk, it has very little saturated fat (see "Saturated Fat Is Bad for Your Heart" on page 29).

Cow's milk has a bit more protein than soy milk, but it's also higher in sugar. And the type of sugar in cow's milk, known as lactose, is hard for many people to digest.

When it comes to vitamin D, it's a draw: Cow's milk and leading brands of soy milk are fortified with the same amount. Both also contain 30 percent of the recommended daily level of calcium. However, the mineral occurs naturally in cow's milk and is added to soy milk. Research funded by Silk shows that the calcium in leading brands of soy milk is just as well absorbed as that in cow's milk.

So what about the effect on bones? While some (but not all) research suggests that plant estrogens in soy, known as isoflavones, may increase bone density, there's much stronger evidence that cow's milk does so. Then again, we don't have solid proof that drinking regular milk actually leads to fewer fractures (see "Milk Is Necessary for Strong Bones" on page 100).

If your concern is cholesterol, research shows that soy protein can lower LDL (bad) cholesterol in people with elevated levels, while the saturated fat in regular milk can increase LDL. But you need at least three glasses of soy milk a day to see any benefit—and it's a small one at that.

While soy milk can be a healthful alternative to regular milk, it doesn't deserve a halo. Those who give it one are just as guilty of jumping to conclusions as I was when I condemned it. But convincing them of that may be tough. When it comes to health foods, sacred cows are hard to slaughter.

Though almonds are a good source of protein, almond milk isn't. An eight-ounce cup has just one gram, compared to about seven grams in soy milk and eight or nine in cow's milk. Rice milk, another alternative to cow's milk, is also low in protein.

MILK IS NECESSARY FOR STRONG BONES

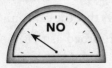 Though I've forgotten much of what I learned in elementary school, I remember just about everything I learned from Schoolhouse Rock. The short musical animations, which aired on Saturday mornings when I was growing up in the 1970s, taught me what a conjunction is, how a bill becomes a law, and what the preamble of the U.S. Constitution says. (I can still recite all the words but only if I sing them to the Schoolhouse Rock tune.)

One of the segments was all about bones. Revealing the "shockeroo" that there's a skeleton under our skin, the video instructed kids how to keep bones strong. "Drinking milk—a glass or two," went the lyrics, "will help your bones to stay in shape and do their job for you."

That's one lesson most viewers probably already knew. From the time we're very young, it's drilled into our heads that everyone needs milk to prevent brittle and broken bones. But here's my own shockeroo: It's not really true.

Randomized studies do show that dairy foods can increase bone density in the short term. But as a whole, research has failed to prove that more dairy leads to fewer fractures, which is what really counts. A meta-analysis of six cohort studies—including one that followed more than 70,000 nurses for 26 years—found that women who drank the most milk had no fewer hip fractures.

What about the notion that milk is a good source of calcium, which we need for strong bones? That's true, but calcium can also come from nondairy natural sources, such as tofu, canned salmon with bones, and leafy green vegetables, as well as fortified products. Though these foods typically contain less calcium than milk, you can still get adequate amounts of the mineral from them.

In countries such as India and Japan, where calcium and dairy intake is low, rates of bone fractures are also relatively low. What this suggests is that bone health is determined by more than how much calcium or dairy we consume. Factors such as genetics, physical activity, body size, and hormone levels also play a role. An especially important contributor, according to research, may be vitamin D. While you can get it from milk, certain kinds of salmon and tuna contain even more. The greatest potential amount comes from sun exposure (see "Most of Us Need More Vitamin D" on page 109).

Some researchers cite the higher fracture rates in milk-guzzling countries as evidence that milk actually weakens bones. Indeed, some studies suggest that a high intake of animal protein (which dairy contains) causes calcium to be pulled from bones and excreted in urine. But in general, research shows that protein doesn't harm bones and may be slightly beneficial.

If you like milk, it's fine to keep drinking it. If you don't, you shouldn't feel compelled to start. Beware of experts who insist that it's hard, if not impossible, to have healthy bones without three servings of dairy a day. Some of these scientists, it turns out, have financial ties to the dairy industry.

That gives me an idea: If they ever produce more Schoolhouse Rock videos, maybe there should be one on critical thinking. I even have the lyrics: *Experts are people too. They have biases like me and you. Before you follow them over the hills, find out who pays their bills.*

Spinach is relatively rich in calcium, but our bodies absorb very little of it. That's because spinach is high in oxalic acid, which binds to calcium and can inhibit absorption. Other leafy green vegetables, such as broccoli, kale, and turnip greens, contain less oxalic acid than spinach and thus are better sources of calcium.

DAIRY PRODUCTS CAUSE CANCER

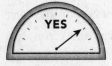 Former New York City mayor Rudy Giuliani and the animal rights group PETA aren't exactly ideological soul mates. But they do have one thing in common: an in-your-face style of combat.

In 2000, the scrappers squared off when PETA used the mayor's image in a billboard ad campaign. Mocking the dairy industry's "Got Milk?" ads, the group showed a forlorn-looking Giuliani with a milk mustache, accompanied by the caption "Got Prostate Cancer?" At the time, the mayor was undergoing treatment for prostate cancer.

When Giuliani threatened to sue, PETA took the billboards down. Nevertheless, the group declared the short-lived campaign a success, saying the controversy had helped raise awareness that dairy products could raise the risk of prostate cancer. Dismissing the alleged danger, Giuliani thumbed his nose at PETA by constantly quaffing milk at public appearances. Perhaps he should have listened to them.

A number of studies have examined the relationship between dairy products and prostate cancer. A meta-analysis of 10 cohort studies, published in the *Journal of the National Cancer Institute*, found that men with the highest intake of dairy products were slightly more likely to develop advanced prostate cancer than those with the lowest intake. In one of these studies, which involved nearly 48,000 health professionals, drinking two or more glasses of milk a day was associated with an increased risk.

Several large cohort studies published since the meta-analysis have identified skim milk and other low-fat dairy products as potential culprits, while exonerating whole dairy. It's not entirely clear why, but some scientists think it may be due to the effects of calcium and vitamin D. Compared to whole milk, nonfat versions have more calcium, which some research suggests may suppress levels of vitamin D in the body. And low levels of vitamin D have been linked to prostate cancer.

Another proposed explanation for the relationship overall is that milk and calcium boost amounts of a hormone called IGF-1, high levels of which are associated with an elevated risk of prostate cancer. A third theory is that estrogen found in milk plays a role.

Prostate isn't the only type of cancer that's been tied to dairy products. So has ovarian cancer, though the evidence overall isn't as strong. If there is an increased risk, researchers suspect it may be due to lactose, the sugar in milk. Lactose is broken down to a sugar called galactose, which studies show could be harmful to cells in the ovaries.

The news is more encouraging when it comes to colorectal cancer. Research has consistently found that drinking lots of milk is associated with a *lower* risk. As for breast cancer, there doesn't appear to be an effect either way.

Still, that didn't stop PETA from including the slogan "Got Breast Cancer?" as part of its "Milk Sucks" campaign. Unlike the prostate cancer ads, these notices featured a pink ribbon instead of a person. That's probably wise. A ribbon is far less likely than Rudy to fight back.

To increase milk production, some cows are injected with the synthetic hormone rBST (recombinant bovine somatotropin), which has been blamed for early puberty in girls. But there's no evidence for this. The hormone is destroyed during pasteurization, and what remains isn't absorbed by the body. Though so-called hormone-free and organic milks are produced without rBST, they still contain small amounts of naturally occurring BST. Studies show that levels of BST in such products are the same as those in milk from rBST-treated cows.

DAIRY PRODUCTS PROMOTE WEIGHT LOSS

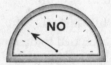 Sometimes advertising messages stick with us long after the ads are gone: Coca-Cola is the "Real Thing," Timex "Takes a Licking and Keeps on Ticking," Kentucky Fried Chicken is "Finger-Lickin' Good."

To that list I would add "Milk Your Diet. Lose Weight!" For years, an array of milk-mustachioed celebrities, ranging from David Beckham to Dr. Phil, urged us to drink milk as a way to slim down. Though the ubiquitous ads were discontinued in 2007, the notion they promoted lives on.

The ads were part of a massive marketing effort by the dairy industry, which also included community events and weight-loss contests with cash prizes. All pushed the message that three daily servings of dairy products could help dieters burn fat and shed extra pounds.

This notion didn't come out of nowhere. Some observational studies had found that people who consumed more calcium—whether through supplements or dairy products—tended to be thinner than those who got less.

Also, several small, short-term studies showed that subjects put on a high-dairy, reduced-calorie diet lost more weight and fat than low-dairy dieters. All were conducted by a dairy-funded researcher at the University of Tennessee who had patented the dairy weight-loss claim and sold licensing rights to the dairy industry.

After other scientists expressed skepticism and consumer activists cried foul with the Federal Trade Commission, the dairy industry decided to suspend its campaign "until further research provides stronger, more conclusive evidence of an association between dairy consumption and weight loss."

Well, there's now further research, including several clinical trials and meta-analyses, and overall it shows no greater weight or fat loss among subjects on high-dairy diets. A few studies have even linked dairy to weight gain.

The Tennessee researcher who got positive results has said that the problem is with everyone else's study designs. Many did not put subjects on a calorie-restricted diet, which he says is necessary for dairy to have an effect. Another shortcoming he cites is that not all participants had a calcium deficiency, something he says is essential for dairy to work its alleged magic. Oh, and add to the list that you must be overweight and not on a high-protein diet.

Such caveats are neither clear nor relevant to most consumers. What the ads said—and what many people continue to hear and believe—is that milk and other dairy products can help you lose weight. Period.

If the ads ever come back, maybe they'll look like those give-aways of cash and cruises with all the fine print:

EAT DAIRY. LOSE WEIGHT!*

*Only if you're overweight and on a calorie-restricted diet that's other-wise too low in calcium and not too high in protein. Restrictions apply. Void where prohibited.

Though dairy's effectiveness against obesity is unproven, it may help prevent two other common problems: type 2 diabetes and high blood pressure. A number of studies have linked consumption of low-fat dairy foods to a reduced risk of both conditions.

Chapter 8

Take (or Leave) Your Vitamins

VITAMIN C FIGHTS COLDS

 Lots of people swear that popping vitamin C pills can keep colds at bay, my mother among them. And they're in good company. The renowned scientist Linus Pauling, two-time winner of the Nobel Prize, championed the idea through popular books in the 1970s. Now, I don't make it a habit of contradicting brilliant scientists—or even worse, my mother—but in this case, I must. After decades of research trying to find proof, the most we can say is that the vitamin may work in a small minority of people and has only a slight effect on symptoms.

In a review by the Cochrane Collaboration, which assesses the scientific evidence for various treatments, researchers pooled data from 29 clinical trials on vitamin C involving more than 11,000 subjects. They found that people taking 200 to 2,000 milligrams (mg) a day were just as likely to catch colds as those who took placebos. But there was an exception: For skiers, soldiers, and marathon runners—people who are exposed to extreme conditions or who push their bodies to the max—the vitamin appeared to cut the risk of colds in half.

So what about the effect on symptoms? Adults who regularly took vitamin C had colds that were shorter, on average, by 8 percent. For children, the decrease was 13 percent. While that may sound impressive, keep in mind that a typical cold lasts 10 days, so those reductions translate to a grand total of about 1 day.

Subjects who started the supplements once they felt sick saw no benefit—unless they took a massive dose of 8,000 mg. That's far more than the 2,000 mg safe upper limit for adults. Above that, vitamin C can cause nausea, indigestion, diarrhea, and kidney stones. Talk about the cure being worse than the disease.

As long as you don't overdo it, there's no evidence that taking vitamin C is harmful. Just keep in mind that the body can absorb only about 500 mg at a time and excretes what it can't use. That means if you take a typical daily dose of 1,000 mg, it's best to split it up. Otherwise, you may be pissing away your investment—literally.

Speaking of cost, beware of high-priced vitamin C brands that promise to provide extra immune protection. It's their sneaky way of claiming to ward off colds without explicitly saying so and running afoul of FDA rules. The truth is that there's no direct evidence that these products are any better than regular vitamin C at fighting colds.

Of course, the best way to get the vitamin is by doing something we've all been told: Eat plenty of fruits and veggies. That's advice from Mom I can't quibble with.

There's evidence that zinc, another common remedy for colds, may be effective. A review by the Cochrane Collaboration found that when taken within 24 hours of the first symptoms, zinc can reduce the severity and length of colds. However, zinc lozenges can cause nausea, and it's not clear what type of zinc or how much is optimal.

MOST OF US NEED MORE VITAMIN D

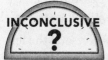

For journalists, it's sometimes surprising what pushes our readers' buttons. Take, for example, a 2010 *New York Times* article that elicited more than 300 online comments, many of them angry. "Boo, hissssss," "absolutely ridiculous," "patent hogwash," and "stupid, false, and a total pack of lies" were typical of the responses. (And, of course, the obligatory "This reporter should be dismissed immediately.")

What riled this virtual mob so much wasn't abortion, the Middle East, or the federal deficit. It was a study on vitamin D. The scientific report, issued by a panel of experts assembled by the Institute of Medicine (IOM), flew in the face of what we've repeatedly heard—that most of us need more vitamin D to protect against an array of conditions.

In fact, many studies do suggest that higher levels of the vitamin might be beneficial. But the history of vitamin supplements such as B, C, E, and beta-carotene—which were initially hailed as lifesavers but then proven ineffective and possibly even harmful in clinical trials—is a good reason for caution until there's more proof.

Doctors have long known that a deficiency of vitamin D can lead to rickets, a bone disorder in children. There's also good evidence from randomized trials that a vitamin D intake of about 800 international units (IU) per day (the current recommendation for people over age 70) reduces the risk of fractures and falls in older people.

As for other benefits, the research is less conclusive. For example, cohort studies have linked low blood levels of vitamin D to a higher risk of heart disease and cardiovascular-related deaths. But there's a dearth of randomized studies on the subject, and the few that have been conducted don't show that vitamin D supplements protect against heart disease or strokes.

For cancer, the science is similarly incomplete. Case-control and cohort research has found an association between low vitamin D levels and an elevated risk of colorectal cancer, but to date, there's no proof from large clinical trials that vitamin D pills can ward off the disease. And while one randomized study did find that women taking vitamin D and calcium had lower rates of breast cancer, cohort studies have generally turned up no link to breast cancer.

Other research raises the possibility that vitamin D could reduce the risk of multiple sclerosis, diabetes, and premature death. But there's also a potential dark side to D: Studies show that people with very high levels are at increased risk of prostate and pancreatic cancer.

So what's the optimal level? The IOM's panel of experts concluded that a blood level of 20 nanograms per milliliter (ng/ml)—a threshold most people now meet—is sufficient to protect bones and that there are not enough hard data to make recommendations about other possible benefits. But other scientists think the magic number is 30 ng/ml or higher—a standard that would require most of us to take a supplement.

There's broader agreement that certain people, including those who are African American, elderly, or obese, or who have limited sun exposure, may need a supplement. That's because their bodies produce less vitamin D, which our skin makes from exposure to sunlight. Foods such as sockeye salmon, tuna, milk, and fortified orange juice are also sources, but getting enough solely through diet is tough.

If you want to hedge your bets and take a supplement, sticking with the recommended daily level—or even exceeding it by several times—appears to be safe. That's good news for those angry responders to the *New York Times* article, many of whom insisted they would keep taking vitamin D no matter what because they're sure it's beneficial. Too bad there's no supplement for overconfidence.

Supplements can be made from two different forms of vitamin D: D_2 (also known as ergocalciferol) and D_3 (cholecalciferol). D_2 is found in plants, while D_3 is the type produced by our bodies. Though the two are often assumed to be equally potent, recent studies show that D_3 may be more effective than D_2 at raising blood levels of the vitamin.

B VITAMINS GIVE YOU ENERGY

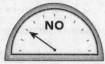

In a classic episode of the 1950s sitcom *I Love Lucy*, Lucy appears in a commercial touting a tonic called Vitameatavegamin. "Are you tired, run down, listless?" she asks. "Do you poop out at parties?" It was a take-off on Geritol, a product heavily promoted in the '50s for its high levels of B vitamins and other nutrients. "If you're feeling tired and listless, weak and run down," said the announcer in one ad, "try Geritol . . . You'll feel better fast."

There are unmistakable echoes of Vitameatavegamin and Geritol in today's ads for "energy" drinks and shots, vitamin supplements, and other products that promise to perk you up. Like the old Geritol, they often contain large doses of B vitamins—sometimes as much as 20,000 percent (no, that's not a typo) of the recommended daily amounts. These vitamins, according to the manufacturers, "support energy production" and "play an important role in energy metabolism."

While that's technically true, it's misleading. We do in fact need certain B vitamins to turn food into energy. But this "energy" is the kind that powers cells in our bodies to do their jobs—not the kind that makes us feel peppy, alert, or able to leap tall buildings in a single bound.

B vitamins can be found in a variety of foods, ranging from beans to bananas to cereal. Though some older people have trouble absorbing B_{12} and need a supplement, most of us easily get sufficient amounts of this and other B vitamins—such as thiamine (B_1), riboflavin (B_2), niacin (B_3), and vitamin B_6—through a normal diet.

There's no proof that exceeding your daily requirement will improve your physical or mental stamina. Studies have found, for example, that giving B vitamins to athletes who are adequately nourished doesn't improve their performance. Likewise, a review of 14 randomized studies concluded that supplements of B_6, B_{12}, and folic acid (B_9) don't improve mental functioning.

For the most part, excess B vitamins simply pass through your body into the toilet. But very high levels of a few—such as B_6, niacin, and folic acid—can cause nerve, liver, or kidney damage. A study of diabetic patients with kidney disease found that taking high-dose B vitamins made their kidney problems worse and increased their odds of heart attacks and strokes.

If B vitamin drinks and supplements do give people a boost, it's likely because of another ingredient they often contain: caffeine. Sometimes it's in the form of substances such as guarana, a tropical plant whose seeds have high levels of caffeine.

In that *I Love Lucy* episode, Vitameatavegamin turns out to be 46 proof. (The old Geritol formulation contained 12 percent alcohol.) Lucy proceeds to get hammered from swallowing one spoonful after another during rehearsals. A modern version of the episode would have her knocking back numerous energy drinks and getting a caffeine high. Somehow it just doesn't seem as funny.

Mixing energy drinks with alcohol, a popular practice among college students, can cause people to underestimate their level of intoxication and impairment. As a result, the combination may increase the risk of injuries more than alcohol alone.

NIACIN IMPROVES CHOLESTEROL LEVELS

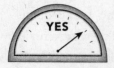

If the B vitamin niacin has an inferiority complex, it's easy to understand why. In recent years, its glamorous cousins vitamins C, D, and E have captured headlines for their alleged powers to save lives, while niacin has been tied to something decidedly less laudable: concealing illegal drug use. The claim, widely circulated on the Internet, is that niacin can help marijuana and cocaine users beat urine drug screenings by clearing the substances from their bodies.

The unseemly allegation, it turns out, is false. But another claim often associated with the vitamin—that it can improve cholesterol readings—is true. And unlike those other vitamins, which often don't live up to their billing, niacin has actually been shown to save lives.

Known officially as vitamin B$_3$ or nicotinic acid, niacin has long been recognized to lower LDL (bad) cholesterol along with blood fats known as triglycerides. But the vitamin's main claim to cholesterol fame, demonstrated in numerous clinical trials, is its ability to raise HDL (good) cholesterol by as much as 35 percent—a benefit no cholesterol medication can match.

Though one large trial found that niacin combined with cholesterol-lowering drugs was no more effective than medication alone in preventing heart attacks, other randomized studies have shown that taking niacin reduces the risk of heart attacks and premature death in people who have heart disease.

To get these benefits, you can't just pop a multivitamin or eat niacin-rich foods, such as chicken breast, beef liver, and peanuts. We're talking about very large doses—as much as three grams a day, which is about 200 times the recommended daily level.

Taking this much can come with some unpleasant side effects, including flushing (burning, tingling, and redness) of the skin, headaches, dizziness, and upset stomach. More serious is the potential for liver damage.

The flushing can be reduced by taking aspirin beforehand, increasing the dose gradually, and using a sustained-release version, which results in slower absorption of the vitamin. However, this form of niacin—sometimes also called timed-release or controlled-release—carries a higher risk of liver problems. You can also find "no flush" supplements, but their active ingredient, inositol hexaniacinate, hasn't been shown to improve cholesterol levels.

High-dose niacin is available with or without a prescription. Even if you use an over-the-counter preparation, it's important to do so under a doctor's care. Otherwise, you could wind up like the folks who've tried taking the vitamin to cheat on drug tests and landed in the emergency room with life-threatening side effects. Maybe it's niacin's way of striking back at those who mistreat the underappreciated nutrient—a vitamin version, you might say, of *Revenge of the Nerds*.

High doses of niacin boost blood levels of the amino acid homocysteine, which when elevated may increase the risk of heart disease. In contrast, other B vitamins (B_6, B_{12}, and folic acid) lower homocysteine levels. However, taking these vitamins has not been shown to prevent heart attacks or strokes.

ANTIOXIDANTS ARE GOOD FOR YOUR EYES

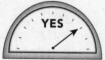

Like vampires, some nutrition myths are hard to kill.

One is the old saw that eating carrots improves your eyesight. During World War II, British officials helped ensure this falsehood's survival by invoking it to explain the Royal Air Force's success at shooting down Nazi bombers. The British pilots were said to have extraordinary night vision because they consumed copious amounts of carrots. It turns out the story was a ruse to keep the Germans from figuring out the real reason for the Brits' superior skill: new technology known as radar.

It's true that a deficiency of vitamin A (which the body makes from beta-carotene in carrots and other foods) can impair vision. However, carrots won't enhance your eyesight if you get enough of the vitamin, which most Americans do through a normal diet. Nevertheless, the carrot myth is alive and well, and now it has a companion: the claim that beta-carotene and other antioxidants in foods and supplements help fight eye problems. I'm pleased to say that we don't need to drive a stake through the heart of this one. It actually has merit.

The strongest evidence is for age-related macular degeneration (AMD), a leading cause of blindness. In a randomized trial sponsored by the National Eye Institute, people with intermediate or advanced AMD who took high-dose antioxidant supplements (consisting of vitamins C and E, beta-carotene, plus zinc) were less likely to experience vision loss and progression of their disease than those who got a placebo.

However, the study also found that antioxidants did not prevent or slow the progression of cataracts. While the results of most other cataract trials involving supplements have been similarly disappointing, cohort studies looking at food have yielded more positive results. As a whole, they show that people who eat diets rich in vitamin C, vitamin E, and beta-carotene have a lower risk of developing cataracts. The same is true of those with high intakes of lutein and zeaxanthin, two antioxidants found in leafy green vegetables such as kale, spinach, and collard greens.

Scientists theorize that antioxidants protect the eyes by neutralizing free radicals, which can result from sunlight exposure and smoking (among other things) and cause damage.

While there's no evidence that antioxidants from food can cause harm, supplements are another story: Beta-carotene is associated with an increased risk of lung cancer among smokers, and vitamin E has been tied to heart failure in people at high risk for cardiovascular disease. What's more, both beta-carotene and vitamin E supplements have been linked to slightly elevated odds of premature death.

Unless you have AMD and it's at the stage where supplements have been shown to be beneficial, your best bet is to stick with antioxidant-rich foods such as cantaloupe, oranges, almonds, kale—and yes, carrots. Just don't count on them to help you see enemy fighters in the dark. If that's your goal, you might be better off consulting a vampire. I hear they have excellent night vision.

Eating large amounts of carrots, sweet potatoes, or other foods high in beta-carotene can turn skin yellowish orange. The discoloration isn't considered dangerous and goes away with reduced intake.

MULTIVITAMINS KEEP YOU HEALTHY

 Have I got a deal for you: an auto insurance policy that will cover everything from oil changes to major body damage. And it costs only pennies a day! Sound good? Just sign here. What, you're puzzled because we almost never pay out claims? Don't let that worry you. You've heard nasty rumors that our company-approved auto-body shops steal customers' hubcaps? Disregard that. No one has proven it . . . yet.

Unless you're someone who obliges those email requests from Nigerians to forward your bank account information, you'd probably run away from this offer. Yet it's analogous to what we get with multivitamins, which millions of people have no qualms about taking.

Multivitamins are widely regarded as an insurance policy to keep us healthy in case our diets aren't sufficient to do the job. The problem is that this insurance has never been shown conclusively to provide benefits for most people, and there are hints it could cause harm.

Though a few studies have linked multivitamin use to a lower risk of heart disease or cancer, most cohort studies have turned up no benefits. For example, the well-designed Women's Health Initiative study, which followed 162,000 postmenopausal women for eight years, found that multivitamin users had no lower rates of heart attacks, strokes, cancer, or premature death.

When a panel of experts appointed by the National Institutes of Health reviewed data from randomized trials, they concluded that the evidence is insufficient to recommend the use of multis to prevent cancer and other chronic diseases in adults. Several clinical trials in older people have also shown that multivitamins don't reduce rates of colds or other infections.

As for possible risks, a large cohort study published in the *Journal of the National Cancer Institute* found that men who took multivitamins more than seven times a week were more likely than nonusers to develop advanced prostate cancer and to die from the disease. Other research has also linked multivitamin use to prostate cancer.

Further, a few studies raise the possibility that large amounts of folic acid, one of the ingredients in multis, could increase the risk of breast cancer. Some scientists are concerned that when you combine the dose in a typical multivitamin with the amount we get from food—all enriched grain products in the United States are required to be fortified with folic acid to prevent birth defects—it could be enough to do harm.

The evidence for this is far from definitive, but it's a reminder that we shouldn't think of multivitamins in isolation. Many foods from cereals to juices contain added nutrients, which essentially make them vitamin supplements too. While vitamin and mineral deficiencies undoubtedly pose a health risk, so can excesses—and if we're not careful, taking multis can cause us to get more than we need.

Multivitamins may make sense for those in special need of a nutrient boost—vegans, people on a very low calorie diet, and women who are pregnant or may become pregnant, for example. But no amount of insurance can make up for a lousy diet. If you believe it can, I've got the perfect homeowners policy to sell you. It provides full coverage in the event of Armageddon. No questions asked!

Beware of multivitamins that supposedly have special benefits, such as boosting immunity, promoting weight loss, or helping your heart. Such claims are marketing gimmicks with little grounding in sound science. In some cases, the products contain added ingredients (such as ginkgo for memory) whose effectiveness is unproven or whose dose is too low to be effective. In others, the multis play up the powers of particular vitamins based on limited evidence.

Chapter 9

Safe *and* Sound?

BAGGED SALAD SHOULD BE WASHED

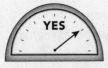

For sellers of packaged fruits and veggies, I possess a highly prized trait: I'm lazy. To avoid cutting, peeling, and washing, I'm willing to shell out extra bucks for apples that are sliced, celery that's diced, carrots that are cut, and pineapple that's cubed.

As for salad, it's bagged lettuce all the way. And, apparently, I'm not alone. Despite its relatively high price, precut salad is a big seller in supermarkets. The packages tell us that the lettuce is "prewashed," "thoroughly washed," "triple washed," or "ready to eat." For kitchen slackers like me, it's a good excuse to avoid spending the 120 seconds it would take to wash and dry the lettuce.

But many people, spooked by recalls and reports of illness tied to bagged salad, take no chances and wash their lettuce. It turns out they have the right idea—though not for the reasons you might think.

In recent years, contaminated bagged lettuce has led to outbreaks of *E. coli* that have sickened hundreds of people and caused several deaths. Health officials can't pinpoint the source of the contamination, but possibilities include birds, water runoff from nearby cattle farms, or cutting utensils used in the field.

When lettuce from different farms is combined—as is customary with bagged salad—and even a small amount of contaminated lettuce gets in the mix, the effects can be far-reaching. Entire batches and multiple bags can end up unsafe to eat. The chlorinated cleaning solution typically used to wash bagged lettuce can kill organisms on the leaves' surfaces, but it doesn't eliminate *E. coli* that's been taken up into the plant. (Some manufacturers have recently switched to an acid solution that they claim is more effective at killing bacteria.) Washing at home won't do the trick either.

Still, a thorough rinsing can remove dirt and germs that remain on the surface after the manufacturer's cleaning process, which evidence suggests isn't foolproof. In a study of more than 200 prewashed lettuce samples, *Consumer Reports* found that a sizable number had high levels of coliform and *Enterococcus* bacteria. (Samples that included spinach and those less than six days from their use-by date tended to fare worst.) While these organisms are unlikely to cause illness, it's an indicator that bagged lettuce isn't quite as clean as those packages would have us believe.

It's not necessary to use a commercial produce wash; research shows that running water is just as effective. Make sure your hands, along with any surfaces that the lettuce touches, are clean. Dry it with a paper towel or spinner when you're done.

Some scientists also recommend soaking your lettuce in vinegar and water, but they admit it's probably too time-consuming for most people. Needless to say, it's a step I'll be skipping.

Like bagged lettuce, baby carrots in bags are washed in a solution of chlorine and water. But contrary to an email rumor, the chlorine doesn't pose a health risk. Nor is it true that the whitening you sometimes see on refrigerated carrots is due to chlorine. It's the harmless result of peeled carrots losing moisture as they're exposed to air.

BOTTLED WATER IS SAFER THAN TAP WATER

 Working out at my gym during peak hours is a little like parking at the mall during Christmas: The law of the jungle rules. If a machine that you want becomes available, you have to pounce before someone else does. But there's one piece of equipment that I never need to fight over: the water fountain. I'm about the only one who ever uses it.

Thanks to bottled water, fountains seem to be going the way of phone booths and typewriters. In 2009, Americans averaged about 28 gallons of bottled water a year—nearly five times the amount consumed two decades earlier. While people often drink bottled water because of the convenience or taste, surveys show another big reason is the perception that it's safer than what comes from the tap. In the vast majority of communities, though, that notion doesn't hold water.

Judging from the ads, you'd think that all bottled water comes from glaciers or pristine mountain springs. In fact, the source is often municipal water supplies of places like Detroit or Wichita—in other words, the tap. Before bottling it, companies typically distill the water or put it through a cleaning process such as deionization or reverse osmosis. Though this may improve the taste, it generally isn't necessary for health reasons, since most tap water is already clean and safe.

Nor does it guarantee that the water is totally free of chemicals or other contaminants. In a 2008 study by the Environmental Working Group—a nonprofit advocacy organization—10 brands of bottled water were found to contain more than three dozen different chemical pollutants. Though it's unclear whether the detected levels pose a health risk, the findings undercut bottled water's reputation for 100 percent purity.

Similarly, a study by researchers in Cleveland revealed that bacteria levels in bottled water varied much more widely than those in local tap water. While most of the 57 bottled water samples tested were at or below the bacteria levels found in tap water, one quarter of the samples had counts that were at least 10 times higher.

The study also found that only 5 percent of the bottled water had optimal levels of fluoride for preventing tooth decay, while 100 percent of the tap water samples did.

Tap water, which is regulated by the Environmental Protection Agency, must undergo frequent testing by certified labs, and consumers must receive regular reports about what's in their water. There are no such requirements for bottled water.

In the last few years, sales of bottled water have slowed thanks to environmental concerns and hard economic times, which have prompted more consumers to think twice about paying for something they can get for free. Evidently, the trend hasn't filtered down to my gym, and I'm hoping it won't. I don't mind sharing the treadmills, but I'd prefer to keep the water fountain to myself.

Contrary to widely circulated Internet rumors, freezing plastic water bottles doesn't release toxic chemicals, and drinking water from a bottle left in a hot car doesn't cause breast cancer. What's more, reusing bottles isn't dangerous as long as you thoroughly wash them by hand after each use to get rid of germs.

MICROWAVING IN PLASTIC IS DANGEROUS

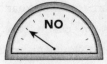 For some reason, microwave ovens seem to be a popular topic for false email rumors. My favorite is the story about the little old lady who supposedly tried to dry off her wet dog by sticking it in the microwave. Sadly, the poor pooch exploded.

A less preposterous—though more pernicious—message concerns the dangers of microwaving food in plastic. The email has spread so rapidly and widely that it's become a nagging concern in kitchens across America.

The gist of the warnings is that heating plastic containers in the microwave releases cancer-causing chemicals called dioxins into food. One version also sounds alarms about plastic wrap, saying that when heated it "drips poisonous toxins into the food."

In fact, there are no dioxins in microwavable plastic containers. Now it's true that a common form of plastic known as polyvinyl chloride (PVC) can generate dioxins when incinerated. But microwavable plastics are not typically made of PVC, and even if PVCs are microwaved, the temperatures aren't hot enough to produce dioxins.

As for other chemicals, plastic containers and wraps contain substances called plasticizers, which make them more flexible. The most common type of plasticizers, known as phthalates, have raised safety concerns because of preliminary research linking them to reproductive abnormalities. However, plastic wraps and containers sold in the United States do not contain phthalates. The kinds of plasticizers they do contain can leach into foods—especially fatty ones—during heating (and also at cooler temperatures), but there's little evidence that the levels to which we're exposed pose a health risk.

To play it safe, though, keep plastic wrap from touching your food during microwaving. If nothing else, this will ensure that melted plastic doesn't wind up as an ingredient in your chicken casserole. Also, stick with containers that are labeled "microwave safe." This means they have been tested according to FDA rules and won't melt or explode. Further, if they release any chemicals during heating, the levels must be 100 times or more below those known to cause harm in lab animals.

The packaging that frozen dinners come in is microwave safe as long as you don't use it more than once. But be careful about plastic foam containers that come from restaurants. Many take-out containers are not designed for the microwave, and zapping them could turn your leftovers into a big melted mess.

Speaking of which, there's an ending to the apocryphal exploding dog tale: The distraught owner sued the oven manufacturer for failing to provide warnings and was awarded millions of dollars. No word on whether the dog had been wrapped in plastic.

Water heated in a microwave oven beyond the boiling point (a phenomenon known as superheating) can explode and cause injuries. Most often this occurs when the water is boiled in a clean cup and then stirred or jostled. Adding something to the water, such as a tea bag, a stir stick, or coffee, during microwaving greatly reduces the risk.

CHEMICALS IN FRENCH FRIES CAUSE CANCER

 If, like me, you have trouble resisting French fries, try visiting a fast-food restaurant in California. Here's what you may find posted on the wall: "Certain foods or beverages sold here, including French fries . . . may contain acrylamide, a chemical known to the state of California to cause cancer." Seeing that will kill your appetite for fries faster than you can say *supersize*.

The warning is there because under California law, companies must notify the public about any cancer-causing chemicals in products they sell. When the state sued food chains for failing to do so, they agreed to post the notices. But the warnings overstate the certainty of the science. While the chemical in question, acrylamide, has generated scary headlines, studies are mixed as to whether eating food containing it really poses a health risk.

Acrylamide is produced when starchy foods such as potatoes are heated to high temperatures. French fries and potato chips have the highest levels, but the chemical is also found in coffee, cereal, crackers, cookies, and bread, among other things. By some estimates, more than one third of the calories we consume come from foods that contain acrylamide.

The chemical is used for industrial production as well, and research shows that exposure to large amounts can lead to neurological problems in workers. In addition, there's evidence that it causes cancer in rodents. But levels fed to animals were at least 1,000 times greater than what we get from food every day, making it hard to extrapolate the findings to people.

Case-control research has found a link between higher exposure levels and estrogen-related breast cancer in postmenopausal women. On the other hand, two large cohort studies have shown that women with the highest intake of acrylamide had no greater risk of breast cancer.

One of those studies, known as the Netherlands Cohort Study, also found an elevated risk of kidney cancer among people consuming the most acrylamide. There were associations with ovarian and endometrial cancers as well, but another large cohort study of Swedish women detected no such risks.

One possible reason for the inconsistencies is that it's hard to accurately measure acrylamide intake. Levels in a particular food can vary widely, depending on how it's processed, cooked, and stored. For example, in FDA tests of McDonald's fries from seven locations, amounts ranged from 155 to 497 parts per billion—a more than threefold difference.

Frying produces the most acrylamide, while boiling, steaming, and microwaving typically form none. Longer cooking times—for example, toasting bread until it blackens or frying potatoes until they're brown—boost levels as well.

If you're concerned, the best way to reduce your exposure is to avoid tobacco smoke, which is a bigger source of acrylamide than food. As for French fries, you won't see a warning in any restaurant that eating them too often can lead to obesity, high blood pressure, heart disease, or diabetes. But that's a far more compelling reason to skip them than an unproven risk of cancer. Too bad it doesn't always work for me.

Soaking potato slices in water for 15 to 30 minutes before you cook them can reduce acrylamide levels. Storing potatoes in the refrigerator increases levels during cooking.

GENETICALLY MODIFIED FOODS ARE HARMFUL

 The science fiction writer H. G. Wells is credited with accurately predicting all kinds of things, from automatic doors to wireless communication to biological warfare. Some would add to that list the horrors of genetically modified foods.

In his 1904 novel *The Food of the Gods and How It Came to Earth*, Wells wrote about an experimental food, cooked up by scientists, called Herakleophorbia IV. When it's fed to chicks, they grow to gargantuan sizes. Other creatures get access to the food, and next thing you know there are giant rats, wasps, and worms terrorizing the population. Then children consume the stuff and become 40 feet tall. I won't give away the ending, but as you might guess, it's not a happy one.

Fortunately, we have no reports of oversize chickens or children due to genetically modified (GM) foods. While critics say that the foods, which they dub "Frankenfoods," could pose health risks, years of testing and widespread use have turned up no solid evidence of harm.

In the United States, most processed foods—such as cereal, chips, and salad dressing—contain GM ingredients, which are created by taking genes from one organism and transferring them to another. Most often this is done to protect crops against pests or herbicides, allowing farmers to use fewer chemicals and get greater yields. For example, most corn grown in the United States is genetically modified to contain a gene from bacteria called Bt, which makes the plants resistant to harmful insects, such as the European corn borer.

While genetic modification may sound unnatural, farmers have essentially been doing it for centuries by crossbreeding plants to create hybrids with particular traits. What's different is that genes in GM foods may come from nonplant sources.

Critics of the practice worry that it might trigger allergic reactions. In a frequently cited example, tests found that soybeans containing a protein from Brazil nuts had the potential to cause reactions in people with nut allergies. As a result, the beans were never put on the market.

In another case, GM corn called StarLink, which was approved only as animal feed because of its potential to cause allergic reactions in people, accidentally got into taco shells. When the shells were recalled, several dozen people reported that they had experienced adverse effects after eating corn-containing products. But an investigation by the Centers for Disease Control and Prevention (CDC) couldn't confirm that the reactions were due to the GM corn. StarLink is no longer grown, and no other GM foods on the market have been proven to cause allergic reactions.

Another concern is that genetic engineering could make some foods toxic. One published study, for example, found intestinal problems in rats that were fed genetically modified potatoes. But the research has been widely criticized by scientists, who say it was poorly designed. A review of this and other research turned up no solid proof of toxicity from GM foods but also noted that there have been no long-term studies.

Of course, there's always the possibility of unintended consequences. GM crops could, in theory, inadvertently crossbreed with other plants, creating hard-to-kill weeds or other undesirable plants. Likewise, GM animals such as salmon could escape their pens and upset the ecosystem. It's one reason the FDA has been slow to grant approval for GM animals.

Speaking of unintended results, the film version of *The Food of the Gods* flopped at the box office and earned one critic's Golden Turkey Award for Worst Rodent Movie of All Time. While it's debatable whether H. G. Wells was prescient about GM foods and their consequences, it's safe to say he didn't foresee siring a cheesy horror flick.

The FDA doesn't require genetically modified foods to be labeled as such because they contain no different nutrients or ingredients than their conventional counterparts. However, in a 2010 survey, 93 percent of consumers said GM foods should be labeled.

IRRADIATED FOOD IS UNSAFE

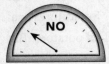 I must admit that I have a mild phobia when it comes to radiation. It's not as though I run away screaming at the site of X-ray machines, but I am a bit uneasy whenever someone aims radiation beams at my body. The fact that my dental hygienist always darts into a lead-enforced bunker while photographing my molars does little to reassure me.

I know I'm not alone, which helps explain why food producers haven't widely embraced the practice of radiating food to kill germs. For many consumers, the prospect of nuked lettuce that glows in the dark is unnerving, if not unappetizing. But in fact, such fears are unfounded.

Food irradiation, which has been around for 100 years, involves using electron beams, gamma-rays, or X rays to kill bacteria and other disease-causing microorganisms. It can also eliminate insects, control the growth of mold, and extend a food's shelf life. The FDA has given its blessing to food irradiation for treating, among other things, meat, poultry, produce, eggs, and spices.

Zapping food does not make it radioactive or expose consumers to radiation. Nor does the process produce radioactive waste. The same technology is widely used to sterilize medical supplies.

Critics say irradiation causes chemical changes in food that can be harmful. As proof, they cite research showing that compounds in irradiated food known as 2-alkylcyclobutanones (2-ACBs) cause DNA damage in cells and promote the development of tumors in rats. However, the doses of 2-ACBs used were 1,000 times greater than levels found in irradiated foods, which makes the relevance of these studies questionable. Further, many other studies of animals fed irradiated foods have failed to turn up any evidence of harm.

Opponents also charge that irradiating food strips it of nutrients. It's true that the process can reduce levels of certain vitamins (especially thiamine), but the losses aren't great enough to matter. Any changes in taste or texture are also minimal in foods that are approved for irradiation.

Then there's the fear that irradiation will become a substitute for proper sanitation and give food producers and government regulators an excuse to be more lax about food safety. Maybe, but these concerns are hypothetical, and the risks from contaminated food are very real, as evidenced by the steady stream of news reports of people seriously sickened by everything from burgers to bagged lettuce (see "Bagged Salad Should Be Washed" on page 121).

While irradiation is by no means a panacea—it doesn't kill harmful viruses, for example, and can't be used on all foods—the CDC estimates that if half the meat and poultry consumed in the United States were irradiated, we could avoid 900,000 cases of foodborne illness, 8,500 hospitalizations, and 350 deaths every year.

Irradiated foods must carry a symbol (known as a radura) showing a flower inside a circle. Maybe instead there should be someone inside the circle puking from food poisoning with a red slash through it. I know it's a bit graphic (okay, gross), but it's likely to make us radiation-phobes forget our fears.

Foods past their "sell by" or "best if used by" dates are not necessarily unsafe to eat. A *sell-by* date tells retailers when to remove the product from shelves. You should buy the food before that date, but it's often fine to use afterward. For example, milk may be okay for five days or so, and eggs for three to five weeks after purchase. A *best-if-used-by* date indicates when the product may start losing flavor or nutritional value.

Chapter 10

Diet Doctrines

VEGETARIAN DIETS ARE MORE HEALTHFUL THAN OTHER DIETS

Nineteenth-century diet crusader Sylvester Graham was not a fan of sex. Believing that it caused debilitation, he advocated a vegetarian diet as one way to keep sexual urges in check. Graham was therefore probably spinning in his grave when some of his vegetarian heirs tried to run a TV ad during the 2009 Super Bowl claiming that vegetarians have better sex.

The commercial, produced by the animal rights group PETA, depicted scantily clad models deriving, uh, pleasure from pumpkins, asparagus, and broccoli stalks. (And I don't mean by eating them.) NBC refused to air the ad, saying it was too sexually explicit. Apparently, the censors missed all those Viagra commercials and, for that matter, many of the shows on the network.

Questions of taste aside, the ad had a major shortcoming: It wasn't true. There's no direct evidence that vegetarians have superior sex lives. As for the claim by PETA and others that going meatless is more healthful, it does have merit—sort of.

Much of what we know about vegetarians' health comes from cohort studies involving subjects in Great Britain and Germany as well as Seventh-Day Adventists in California. The research consistently shows that vegetarians tend to be leaner than nonvegetarians and have lower rates of heart disease. They also appear to have a lower risk of diabetes.

Concerns that vegetarian diets lead to protein and iron deficiencies are largely unfounded. The same goes for fears that they weaken bones: Research shows that vegetarians have no greater risk of fractures if they consume enough calcium. While it can be harder for vegetarians (especially those who avoid all animal products) to get adequate amounts of calcium, vitamin B_{12}, and certain other nutrients, it is possible with proper planning.

Whether vegetarian diets are better for you depends on what they're compared to. For example, British studies show that vegetarians have lower cancer rates overall than meat eaters but not lower than fish eaters. Likewise, vegetarians tend to live longer than those who eat a standard Western diet, but they don't outlive health-conscious people who are not vegetarians.

Which raises another question: Are vegetarians healthier mainly because of their diets or because of their overall lifestyles, which tend to be healthier than average? Teasing out these factors is tricky.

Yet another challenge is defining exactly what we mean by

vegetarian. Beyond shunning meat, vegetarians vary in what they eat, and lumping them all together can be misleading. A vegetarian whose diet consists largely of beans and vegetables, for example, isn't exactly the same as one who lives on doughnuts and French fries.

You can find vegetarians who consume nothing derived from animals (known as vegans), as well as those who eat fish (pesco-vegetarians) and poultry (pollo-vegetarians). There are also vegetarians whose diets include eggs (ovo-vegetarians), dairy (lacto-vegetarians), and both eggs and dairy (ovo-lacto-vegetarians).

And let's not forget those models in the PETA ad, whose patterns of vegetable use fall into yet another category. I'm not sure what they're called. Sexegetarians, perhaps?

Animal sources of protein contain all nine essential amino acids (meaning those our bodies can't make), while plant foods typically lack one or more amino acids. That's why people who avoid animal products need to consume so-called complementary proteins from various plant sources, such as beans, nuts, and rice. But contrary to previous advice, these foods don't have to be eaten at the same time.

A MEDITERRANEAN DIET IS GOOD FOR YOU

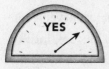

Ready for a *Jeopardy!* challenge? Here's the answer: The Mediterranean diet shares this with Chinese calligraphy, woodcrafting in Madagascar, and polyphonic singing by African Pygmies. The correct question . . . coming up.

Despite what many of us would like to believe, the Mediterranean diet does not consist of Domino's Pizza and Chef Boyardee ravioli. Instead, it refers to what people in Crete, southern Italy, and surrounding areas ate 50 years ago: large amounts of vegetables, fruits, beans, nuts, seeds, whole grains, and olive oil; a few servings a week of fish, poultry, and eggs; low to moderate amounts of dairy products; very little red meat; and, of course, wine with meals.

Over the years, the Mediterranean diet has been the subject of countless studies, and the near-unanimous verdict is that it appears to be good for us—in a number of ways. Pooling data from 18 cohort studies that collectively followed more than two million people, researchers found that the diet is associated with a reduced risk of developing and dying from heart disease, stroke, cancer, Alzheimer's disease, and Parkinson's disease. Moreover, people following the diet have lower overall rates of premature death.

There's also solid evidence from experimental studies. In a randomized clinical trial known as the Lyon Diet Heart Study, heart attack patients were instructed to follow either a Mediterranean diet or a so-called prudent diet recommended by the American Heart Association. Over the next four years, those in the Mediterranean diet group had fewer subsequent heart attacks and heart-related deaths.

Other randomized trials have shown the diet to have beneficial effects on cholesterol, blood pressure, blood glucose, insulin, and inflammation in arteries (which can contribute to heart disease). In addition, several experimental studies have found that it can help promote weight loss.

So which parts of the Mediterranean diet are most responsible for its apparent benefits? The vegetables? The olive oil? The red wine? Though some researchers have tried to pinpoint the magic ingredient(s), we can't say for sure. Scientists suspect the key is people's overall eating patterns rather than individual components of the diet. In fact, there's not even a single, standard definition of a Mediterranean diet. Those who follow it don't eat exactly the same foods, yet they consistently seem to benefit.

Ironically, as more Americans are trying to go Mediterranean, residents of that region have been abandoning their own diet for American-style fare of fast food, soda, chips, and candy. And they're paying a heavy price: Obesity rates among children in Greece, for example, have been rising rapidly.

Which brings us back to our *Jeopardy!* challenge. Here's the correct question: What is . . . the United Nation's list of cultural traditions in need of protection? Thanks to aggressive lobbying by Italy, UNESCO has added the Mediterranean diet to its official Intangible Cultural Heritage list. Did you get it right? If so, you win a prize! Treat yourself to a heaping plate of fresh vegetables sautéed in olive oil.

People in Mediterranean countries often eat dinner late in the evening, a practice that some diet regimens forbid because it supposedly leads to weight gain. Though a few preliminary studies provide some support for this claim, research overall has failed to prove it. It's true that our metabolism slows down when we sleep (which is a main reason for the don't-eat-after-8-p.m. rule), but we still continue to burn calories.

DETOX DIETS MAKE YOU HEALTHIER

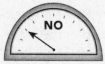

At the peak of the British Empire, the monarchy reigned over a quarter of the globe's inhabitants. Today, it's a small fraction of that. With less to do these days, the royals presumably have some extra time on their hands. Prince Charles has come up with at least one way to fill it: peddling herbal detox products.

The Prince of Wales, heir to the throne, sells a tincture made from extracts of artichoke and dandelion, which are touted as "cleansing and purifying herbs to help support the body's natural elimination and detoxification processes." It's one of a number of products offered by Duchy Originals, a company formed by His Royal Highness to promote organic farming and holistic health. Proceeds go to charity.

On this side of the pond, our version of royalty, Oprah Winfrey, has also embraced dietary detox, as have celebrities such as Gwyneth Paltrow, Demi Moore, and Angelina Jolie. Detox regimens are touted as a way to boost energy, lose weight, prevent chronic conditions, and improve overall health by flushing out toxins that build up inside the body. Despite the high-profile endorsements, there's no hard evidence that the diets do any good; indeed, they have the potential to cause harm.

Detox diets typically eliminate certain foods and severely restrict calories, while prescribing juices and other liquids—and sometimes laxatives and supplements—that allegedly have detoxifying effects. For example, on Master Cleanse, aka the Lemonade Diet, you live for 10 days on salt water and a concoction of lemon juice, water, maple syrup, and cayenne pepper, along with laxative tea. The Martha's Vineyard Diet Detox gets you to guzzle up to 40 ounces of herbal tea, 16 ounces of vegetable-based soup, and 32 ounces of green juice every day. Herbal cleansing supplements and weekly coffee enemas are also encouraged.

Though detox diet promoters claim that our insides, like house pipes, require periodic cleaning, that's not the case. Our liver, lungs, kidneys, colon, and skin are constantly removing harmful substances, and they're more than up to the task for most people. Even if our bodies did need help eliminating toxins, there's no evidence that detox diets could provide it.

Nevertheless, some people swear that the diets make them feel more energetic or even euphoric. One reason could be that they're experiencing starvation, which can have this effect. Another is that they're cutting out things like junk food, alcohol, and excess calories, which make us feel sluggish.

As for the promise of weight loss—the main reason many people try detox diets—any extremely low-calorie regimen can help you shed pounds. But they're likely to be quickly regained once you go off the diet.

Contrary to what proponents will tell you, symptoms such as headaches, fatigue, pain, or cravings are not signs that a detox diet is working. Repeated or prolonged detox dieting can potentially lead to vitamin and mineral deficiencies, muscle breakdown, and blood sugar problems. Chronic use of laxatives can be especially harmful.

Another potential danger is the implicit message that it's okay to overindulge as long as you undergo periodic "cleansings." It's one reason that a British professor of complementary medicine has taken Prince Charles to task for his tincture. Accusing him of relying on "make believe and superstition," the doctor has denounced his future king's product as "outright quackery." He probably shouldn't count on an invitation to the next coronation or royal wedding.

Wheatgrass juice, a common ingredient in detox diets, is touted for its ability to cleanse the body and treat or prevent a wide array of conditions, including diabetes and cancer. But there's little evidence that wheatgrass has any health benefits beyond those of other green plant foods such as spinach.

A CAVEMAN DIET IS IDEAL

As a collector of cartoons, I seem to come across two subjects fairly often: eating and cave dwelling. Sometimes you find the topics together, as in one cartoon that shows a caveman heading out with spear in hand. Standing in the doorway is his wife, who calls after him, "Try to kill something that will allow me to stay within a daily 1,800 calorie diet."

For some folks, combining prehistoric living with modern dieting is no joke. They're followers of the so-called Caveman Diet, also known as the Paleo or Stone Age Diet, which is based on what people are presumed to have eaten before the emergence of agriculture 10,000 years ago.

The diet includes foods our ancestors could have hunted or

gathered, such as lean meat, fish, eggs, vegetables, fruits, and nuts. It prohibits things not available to them, such as dairy products, grains, legumes, salt, and sugar.

The rationale is that human beings aren't genetically designed to eat much of what we put into our bodies today. Nature intended us to follow a prehistoric diet, the theory goes, and our failure to do so has led to the epidemics of obesity, heart disease, diabetes, and other chronic conditions.

As evidence, proponents cite the experiences of societies that have stuck closely to this dietary ideal. One is the tropical island of Kitava, part of Papua New Guinea, where studies show that modern maladies are rare. However, it's impossible to know for certain whether this is due to the Kitavans' diet or some other aspect of their lifestyle.

Several small, short-term studies have measured the effects of a Caveman Diet in Western populations. In one, nine overweight subjects who were put on the diet for 10 days experienced improvements in blood pressure, cholesterol, and glucose tolerance (a measure of how well the body handles sugar). In others involving people with diabetes or prediabetes, a Caveman Diet resulted in better glucose tolerance than a Mediterranean diet and more favorable readings for blood pressure, good cholesterol, and weight than a standard diabetes diet.

Though the research is too preliminary to permit any firm conclusions, it does appear that the diet's embrace of fruits, veggies, and nuts, along with its avoidance of sweets, refined grains, and junk food, makes it healthful overall. But there's little evidence that shunning whole grains, beans, or dairy is necessary for optimal health.

Nor is there proof that eating lots of meat, as many of the diet's adherents do, is beneficial, and it could be harmful (see "Red Meat Is Bad for You" on page 80). The wild beasts that cavemen killed and consumed are a far cry from what we get at the supermarket— even if it's organic, free-range, and grass-fed.

In truth, we can't be sure what cavemen ate, which is a problem with the whole concept. Based on what anthropologists do know, prehistoric diets varied widely depending on where people lived and what was available to them. Whatever they ate, their health wasn't exactly ideal—a point made by a *New Yorker* cartoon that shows two cavemen puzzling over something. "Our air is clean, our water is pure, we all get plenty of exercise, everything we eat is organic and free-range," says the caption, "and yet nobody lives past thirty."

Some advocates of food-combining diets claim that our bodies are not designed to digest certain types of foods together. For example, these regimens often include eating fruit by itself; otherwise, the food will allegedly rot in the stomach. There's no sound scientific basis for this notion or for food combining in general. The human digestive system is quite capable of handling all kinds of foods, regardless of whether we eat them separately or together.

DIETS HIGH IN WATERY FOODS HELP YOU LOSE WEIGHT

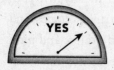

Jessica Seinfeld, the wife of the comedian, has a solution to the perennial challenge of getting kids to eat vegetables: trick them. In her books, she shows parents of picky eaters how to take pureed veggies and sneak them into familiar foods like macaroni and cheese, chicken nuggets, and brownies.

In what sounds like a plot from a *Seinfeld* episode, scientists have tried the same trick on adults to help them lose weight, and they're hoping restaurants and food companies will follow their lead. (I can just imagine an episode in which Jerry recoils from some food because he suspects it's spiked with veggies, and Kramer tries to turn the concept into a money-making scheme by growing broccoli in his bathtub.)

Vegetables are high in water, and the idea is to increase people's intake of watery foods so that they fill up without consuming excess calories—essentially eating more to weigh less. As far-fetched as it sounds, this diet—which has been promoted through the media and popular books—may very well be effective.

At the core of the Volumetrics Diet, as it's called, is the notion of energy density, which refers to the number of calories per gram of food. Watery and high-fiber foods such as vegetables, fruits, soups, beans, and nonfat yogurt are low in energy density, while things like cheese, meat, and cookies have a high density.

Human studies in lab settings show that people typically consume about the same volume of food every day. If calories are cut by lowering energy density but the amount of food remains the same, subjects don't feel deprived. For example, in that research where scientists sneaked pureed veggies into entrees to decrease energy density, people reported feeling just as full from these dishes as they did from versions with higher energy densities.

So how does this affect our weight? A cohort study of 50,000 women found that those whose diets increased the most in energy density over the course of eight years gained the most weight. And several randomized studies show that decreasing energy density leads to weight loss. In one of them, which involved 97 obese women, subjects assigned to eat less fat and more water-rich foods shed more pounds after one year than those who just reduced their fat intake. The watery-food group ate more and felt less hungry, which likely made it easier for them to stick to their diets.

Studies show that soup in particular can be effective at filling you up and promoting weight loss. But not just any soup. Broth-based soups such as vegetarian vegetable typically have a much lower energy density than creamy ones like broccoli and cheese, which at some restaurants can tip the scales at more than 500 calories per bowl.

By the way, the classic "Soup Nazi" episode of *Seinfeld*, in which an ill-tempered soup shop owner berates and expels customers for violating his strict ordering procedures, was inspired by a real character. If you ever encounter him in one of his restaurants, I wouldn't suggest grilling him about the energy density of his soups. Just place your order, have your money ready, and step to your left.

As you might expect, watermelons are high in water. But a few vegetables are even higher. Cucumbers, lettuce, celery, and zucchini are at least 95 percent water, compared to 92 percent for watermelon.

VERY LOW CALORIE DIETS EXTEND YOUR LIFE

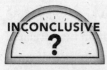

If you're ever invited to a party for the CR Society, you may want to eat before you go. You won't find martinis, meatballs, cheese, or cookies there. Instead, be prepared to dine on flour-free bread, pureed vegetable dip, and seltzer water. You're sure to go away hungry, which is precisely the idea.

CR stands for "calorie restriction." Members of the society believe that severely limiting how much they eat, while squeezing in necessary nutrients, will make them healthier and extend their lives. Indeed, there is proof that starving yourself is beneficial—assuming you're a fly, worm, fish, rodent, or monkey. If you're a person, however, the science is still a few nuggets shy of a Happy Meal.

Animal studies from the past 75 years show that restricting calories by 30 percent can increase lifespan by 30 percent or more. It also prevents or delays conditions such as diabetes, cancer, heart disease, and brain disorders.

Scientists aren't sure why, but they theorize that the benefits may be due to a built-in survival mechanism that makes animals heartier when food is scarce. Decreases in body temperature, insulin, and inflammation that result from calorie restriction are thought to play a role, along with an increased ability to fight harmful free radicals.

In small, preliminary studies of people on low-calorie diets, researchers have found some of these same effects, along with more favorable levels of body fat, blood pressure, and cholesterol than those in people on normal diets.

Other human evidence comes from World War II, when food shortages in Europe were accompanied by a drop in heart-related deaths. CR enthusiasts also point to Okinawa, where people have traditionally consumed Spartan diets. This region of Japan has the longest life expectancy in the world and the highest percentage of centenarians. (This may be changing as more Okinawans gorge on American-style fast food.)

However, none of this adds up to proof that CR extends people's lives, and there's some concern it may do harm. Possible risks include loss of libido, menstrual irregularities, bone thinning, cold sensitivity, slower wound healing, and psychological problems. In addition, studies show that people who are very thin have higher death rates than those who are heavier, though it's unclear whether skinniness itself is responsible.

Even if CR is beneficial and safe, there's the issue of practicality. Unlike rats in a cage, we live in an environment where food is ubiquitous, and constantly suppressing the urge to indulge requires tremendous willpower. A government-funded study called CALERIE is testing the feasibility of a more modest 25 percent reduction in calories, and researchers are working to develop medications that would produce the same benefits as CR without requiring us to forgo enchiladas and ice cream sundaes.

At this point, though, that's still (noncaloric) pie in the sky. If and when such a drug ever comes out, most of us will probably be long gone. Perhaps CR adherents will still be around to celebrate, though. With arugula and green tea, of course.

Fasting may be comparable to calorie restriction in its effects. In studies, animals that are deprived of food every other day, while otherwise allowed to consume as much as they please, reap the same benefits as those on a calorie-restricted diet. Human research is very limited, however, so it's unclear whether fasting on alternate days is beneficial or safe in people.

Conclusion

**TEN TIPS FOR DECIPHERING
DIET AND NUTRITION CLAIMS**

Trying to make sense of the seemingly endless stream of food and nutrition claims can be overwhelming. Remembering the following 10 rules will make the task easier and allow you to stay focused on what's really important:

1. **Don't fixate on particular foods.** Be wary of lists of miraculous "superfoods" you *must* eat or "toxic" foods you should *never* touch. Rather than worrying about squeezing one food or another into your diet, focus on your overall eating patterns, which should include plenty of vegetables, fruits, whole grains, fish, legumes, and good fats, and limited amounts of refined carbohydrates, junk food, red meat, and trans fats.

2. **Look beyond narrow categories like carbs and calories.** Many diet books and seals of approval on foods empha-

size one or two factors, such as the calorie or carbohydrate count, while giving short shrift to other important things, like fiber, sodium, or trans fat. The fact that a hamburger is lower in calories than a salad doesn't necessarily make it a better option. Likewise, just because fruit punch or cereal has added vitamins doesn't mean it's healthful. What's important is the overall nutritional profile. You can get this from comprehensive food-scoring systems such as NuVal, which ranks the healthfulness of foods based on more than 30 factors.

3. **Forget about fad diets.** A plethora of weight-loss plans promise to melt away pounds quickly and easily. But in the long run, they rarely work. About 95 percent of dieters eventually regain lost weight. Instead of searching for the secret to skinniness, which doesn't exist, try to eat more healthfully and be mindful of how much you're consuming. Combined with exercise, this approach can prevent weight gain and, over time, lead to weight loss. And unlike dieting, it's something you can stick with long term.

4. **Recognize the limits of vitamin pills.** While vitamin and mineral supplements can help make up for deficiencies of nutrients, they generally don't live up to their billing when it comes to preventing disease, boosting energy, or improving your overall health. Supplements pack far

less nutritional punch than food, which contains multiple nutrients that interact with one another and with other foods in a variety of complex ways. As a result, vitamin pills can't compensate for an unhealthful diet. And they can cause harm if you take too much of certain nutrients.

5. **Ignore health claims on food packages and in ads.** A few such claims, such as those related to sodium and high blood pressure, are officially approved by the FDA, but most aren't. They fall under a loophole that allows companies to use sneaky language like "helps maintain healthy cholesterol levels" or "helps support a healthy immune system." Because these phrases don't explicitly say that the food prevents or treats disease—even though that's what any normal person would infer—manufacturers don't have to provide any evidence. What's more, there are no strict definitions for frequently used terms such as *all natural*, *low sugar*, and *made with* whole grains or real fruit. Because it's virtually impossible to distinguish between legitimate and misleading claims by manufacturers, the best approach is to disregard them all and get your information from the Nutrition Facts panel on the package.

6. **Don't be swayed by celebrities.** A number of entertainers have authored books pushing particular diet regimens, and the media often report on celebrities' dietary

"secrets." It can be tempting to believe people we admire who are thin, glamorous, and beautiful. But their fame and looks don't make them authorities on nutrition and health. Though celebrities may cite studies and so-called experts to make their case, their approaches can be scientifically baseless and even potentially harmful. Just as you wouldn't look to nutrition experts for entertainment, you shouldn't look to entertainers for nutrition advice.

7. **Verify emails before forwarding them.** The vast majority of emails about food and nutrition are half truths or outright hoaxes. If someone forwards you an email claiming, for example, that canola oil is toxic or that asparagus cures cancer, assume it's not true, no matter how scientific it sounds. Check it out with a reputable source like Snopes.com or Urbanlegends.about.com. Forwarding unconfirmed claims only adds to the hype, misinformation, and confusion.

8. **Don't be influenced by just one study.** When you encounter news reports about the latest study, don't jump to conclusions based on that alone. Remember that it's just one piece of a puzzle. What matters is the big picture—what scientists call the totality of the evidence. For a credible overview of the science, check out online sources such as the Nutrition Source from Harvard School of Public Health, or newsletters such as

Nutrition Action Healthletter, the Tufts Health & Nutrition Letter, and the Berkeley Wellness Letter. Or go to www.pubmed.gov and look up the research yourself.

9. **Learn to live with ambiguity and change.** We all want black and white answers. But that's not always possible when it comes to diet and health. We have to deal with, and distinguish among, various shades of gray. Understanding how different types of studies are conducted makes this much easier. Also, recognize that scientific information isn't set in stone; it's always evolving. This means advice will sometimes change as scientists learn more. Don't let that frustrate you. Instead, embrace the change and alter your eating habits accordingly.

10. **Enjoy eating!** As I said at the beginning of this book, all the admonitions about which foods we should and shouldn't consume can make eating a stressful chore. But it doesn't have to be that way. Using science as your guide, focus on the claims with the greatest credibility and relevance, and tune out the rest. That way, you'll feel less overwhelmed. While following sound nutrition advice is important for good health, it need not spoil your dinner. Bon appétit!

Acknowledgments

Some things are easier the second time around. For me, writing a book proved to be one of them, thanks to the help of so many people.

My literary agent, Lynn Johnston, offered superb guidance that was crucial to transforming a concept into a book. Though *brilliant* is a word that's often used indiscriminately, it definitely applies to Lynn. Her insights and advice were always smart and spot-on.

I'm equally grateful to my editor at Perigee Books, Meg Leder, who skillfully shepherded me through the publishing process, patiently responding to my steady stream of questions and concerns. Her incisive comments strengthened the manuscript, and her unfailing professionalism and cheerfulness made working with her a delight.

Thanks are also due to my outstanding research assistants, Mara Betsch, Kimberly Holland, and Nicole Ferring Holovach, whose help was indispensable. They were able to dig up whatever I needed far more adeptly and efficiently than I ever could have myself.

My colleagues at Everwell, Sean Kelley, Mria Dangerfield, Andrew Spratt, and Tom Morris, served as a valuable sounding board on everything from word selection to cover design. Special thanks to Sean, who saved me when I got stuck by coming up with ingenious angles and helpful information.

My good friend and business partner Loren Goldfarb gave me the benefit of his creative insights and unvarnished opinions. My aunt Doris Califf, who tirelessly promoted my last book, began spreading the word about this one before I even started writing it.

I'm also deeply indebted to Debra Califf, Edward Felsenthal, David Katz, Lisa Lillien, Carolyn O'Neil, Jonathan Ringel, Emily Weaver, Deb Weisshaar, and Amanda Wolf, who took time to read drafts or discuss the manuscript with me and provide invaluable feedback.

My mother, Scottie, managed to plow through several drafts of every chapter, offering both praise (as you'd expect from a mom) and constructive criticism. Since encouraging me to publish a story in a children's magazine when I was nine years old, she's been my number one editor and cheerleader. She has my eternal thanks—and love.

References

INTRODUCTION

Choiniere CJ, Lando A. "2008 Health and Diet Survey." www.fda.gov/Food/Science Research/ResearchAreas/ConsumerResearch/ucm193895.htm.

"False Food Fads Number 39: Physician Gives List of Harmful Diet Doctrines That Have Become Popular." *Washington Post*, April 10, 1910.

Lesser LI, Ebbeling CB, Goozner M, et al. "Relationship Between Funding Source and Conclusion among Nutrition-Related Scientific Articles." *PLoS Medicine* 4 (2007): e5.

1. DRIVEN TO DRINK

Coffee Is Bad for You

Choi HK, Curhan G. "Coffee Consumption and Risk of Incident Gout in Women: The Nurses' Health Study." *American Journal of Clinical Nutrition* 92 (2010): 922–927.

Hallström H, Wolk A, Glynn A, Michaëlsson K. "Coffee, Tea and Caffeine Consumption in Relation to Osteoporotic Fracture Risk in a Cohort of Swedish Women." *Osteoporosis International* 17 (2006): 1055–1064.

Hu G, Bidel S, Jousilahti P, et al. "Coffee and Tea Consumption and the Risk of Parkinson's Disease." *Movement Disorders* 22 (2007): 2242–2248.

Huxley R, Lee CM, Barzi F, et al. "Coffee, Decaffeinated Coffee, and Tea Consumption in Relation to Incident Type 2 Diabetes Mellitus: A Systematic Review with Meta-Analysis." *Archives of Internal Medicine* 169 (2009): 2053–2063.

Lopez-Garcia E, Rodriguez-Artalejo F, Rexrode KM, et al. "Coffee Consumption and Risk of Stroke in Women." *Circulation* 119 (2009): 1116–1123.

Lopez-Garcia E, van Dam RM, Li TY, et al. "The Relationship of Coffee Consumption with Mortality." *Annals of Internal Medicine* 148 (2008): 904–914.

McCusker RR, Fuehrlein B, Goldberger BA, et al. "Caffeine Content of Decaffeinated Coffee." *Journal of Analytical Toxicology* 30 (2006): 611–613.

Savitz DA, Chan RL, Herring AH, et al. "Caffeine and Miscarriage Risk." *Epidemiology* 19 (2008): 55–62.

Weng X, Odouli R, Li DK. "Maternal Caffeine Consumption during Pregnancy and the Risk of Miscarriage: A Prospective Cohort Study." *American Journal of Obstetrics and Gynecology* 198 (2008): 279.

Wu JN, Ho SC, Zhou C, et al. "Coffee Consumption and Risk of Coronary Heart Diseases: A Meta-Analysis of 21 Prospective Cohort Studies." *International Journal of Cardiology* 137 (2009): 216–225.

Yu X, Bao Z, Zou J, Dong J. "Coffee Consumption and Risk of Cancers: A Meta-Analysis of Cohort Studies." *BMC Cancer* 11 (2011): 96.

Red Wine Is the Most Beneficial Type of Alcohol

Barefoot JC, Grønbaek M, Feaganes JR, et al. "Alcoholic Beverage Preference, Diet, and Health Habits in the UNC Alumni Heart Study." *American Journal of Clinical Nutrition* 76 (2002): 466–472.

Cleophas TJ. "Wine, Beer and Spirits and the Risk of Myocardial Infarction: A Systematic Review." *Biomedicine & Pharmacotherapy* 53 (1999): 417–423.

Di Castelnuovo A, Rotondo S, Iacoviello L, et al. "Meta-Analysis of Wine and Beer Consumption in Relation to Vascular Risk." *Circulation* 105 (2002): 2836–2844.

Grønbaek M, Becker U, Johansen D, et al. "Type of Alcohol Consumed and Mortality from All Causes, Coronary Heart Disease, and Cancer." *Annals of Internal Medicine* 133 (2000): 411–419.

Grønbaek M, Deis A, Sørensen TI, et al. "Mortality Associated with Moderate Intakes of Wine, Beer, or Spirits." *BMJ* 310 (1995): 1165–1169.

Klatsky AL, Friedman GD, Armstrong MA, Kipp H. "Wine, Liquor, Beer, and Mortality." *American Journal of Epidemiology* 158 (2003): 585–595.

Mukamal KJ, Conigrave KM, Mittleman MA, et al. "Roles of Drinking Pattern and Type of Alcohol Consumed in Coronary Heart Disease in Men." *New England Journal of Medicine* 348 (2003): 109–118.

Opie LH, Lecour S. "The Red Wine Hypothesis: From Concepts to Protective Signalling Molecules." *European Heart Journal* 28 (2007): 1683–1693.

Rimm EB, Klatsky A, Grobbee D, Stampfer MJ. "Review of Moderate Alcohol Consumption and Reduced Risk of Coronary Heart Disease: Is the Effect Due to Beer, Wine, or Spirits." *BMJ* 312 (1996): 731–736.

Wine Institute. "2009 California Wine Shipments to the U.S. Rise Modestly: Retail Value Falls 3% as Consumers Trade Down." Press release, April 8, 2010.

Alcohol Causes Breast Cancer

Allen NE, Beral V, Casabonne D, et al. "Moderate Alcohol Intake and Cancer Incidence in Women." *Journal of the National Cancer Institute* 101 (2009): 296–305.

Collaborative Group on Hormonal Factors in Breast Cancer. "Alcohol, Tobacco and Breast Cancer—Collaborative Reanalysis of Individual Data from 53 Epidemiological Studies, Including 58,515 Women with Breast Cancer and 95,067 Women without the Disease." *British Journal of Cancer* 87 (2002): 1234–1245.

Key J, Hodgson S, Omar RZ, et al. "Meta-Analysis of Studies of Alcohol and Breast Cancer with Consideration of the Methodological Issues." *Cancer Causes & Control* 17 (2006): 759–770.

Li CI, Chlebowski RT, Freiberg M, et al. "Alcohol Consumption and Risk of Postmenopausal Breast Cancer by Subtype: The Women's Health Initiative Observational Study." *Journal of the National Cancer Institute* 102 (2010): 1422–1431.

Peters R, Peters J, Warner J, et al. "Alcohol, Dementia and Cognitive Decline in the Elderly: A Systematic Review." *Age and Ageing* 37 (2008): 505–512.

Singletary KW, Gapstur SM. "Alcohol and Breast Cancer: Review of Epidemiologic and Experimental Evidence and Potential Mechanisms." *Journal of the American Medical Association* 286 (2001): 2143–2151.

Smith-Warner SA, Spiegelman D, Yaun SS, et al. "Alcohol and Breast Cancer in Women: A Pooled Analysis of Cohort Studies." *Journal of the American Medical Association* 279 (1998): 535–540.

You Need Eight Glasses of Water a Day for Good Health

Altieri A, La Vecchia C, Negri E. "Fluid Intake and Risk of Bladder and Other Cancers." *European Journal of Clinical Nutrition* 57 (2003): S59–S68.

Dennis EA, Flack KD, Davy BM. "Beverage Consumption and Adult Weight Management: A Review." *Eating Behaviors* 10 (2009): 237–246.

Fink HA, Akornor JW, Garimella PS, et al. "Diet, Fluid, or Supplements for Secondary Prevention of Nephrolithiasis: A Systematic Review and Meta-Analysis of Randomized Trials." *European Urology* 56 (2009): 72–80.

Negoianu D, Goldfarb S. "Just Add Water." *Journal of the American Society of Nephrology* 19 (2008): 1041–1043.

Panel on Dietary Reference Intakes for Electrolytes and Water, et al. *Dietary Reference Intakes for Water, Potassium, Sodium, Chloride, and Sulfate*. Washington, DC: National Academies Press, 2005.

"Survey Says: Hydration Trumps Sex." *Cooking Light* (August 2009). www.cookinglight.com/magazine/womens-wellness-poll-00400000054172.

Valtin H. " 'Drink at Least Eight Glasses of Water a Day.' Really? Is There Scientific Evidence for '8 x 8'?" *American Journal of Physiology—Regulatory, Integrative and Comparative Physiology* 283 (2002): R993–R1004.

Wipke-Tevis DD, Williams DA. "Effect of Oral Hydration on Skin Microcirculation in Healthy Young and Midlife and Older Adults." *Wound Repair and Regeneration* 15 (2007): 174–185.

Diet Soda Makes You Fat

Brown RJ, de Banate MA, Rother KI. "Artificial Sweeteners: A Systematic Review of Metabolic Effects in Youth." *International Journal of Pediatric Obesity* 5 (2010): 305–312.

Dhingra R, Sullivan L, Jacques PF, et al. "Soft Drink Consumption and Risk of Developing Cardiometabolic Risk Factors and the Metabolic Syndrome in Middle-Aged Adults in the Community." *Circulation* 116 (2007): 480–488.

Ehlen LA, Marshall TA, Qian F, et al. "Acidic Beverages Increase the Risk of In Vitro Tooth Erosion." *Nutrition Research* 28 (2008): 299–303.

Fowler SP, Williams K, Resendez RG, et al. "Fueling the Obesity Epidemic? Artificially Sweetened Beverage Use and Long-Term Weight Gain." *Obesity* (Silver Spring) 16 (2008): 1894–1900.

Malik VS, Schulze MB, Hu FB. "Intake of Sugar-Sweetened Beverages and Weight Gain: A Systematic Review." *American Journal of Clinical Nutrition* 84 (2006): 274–288.

Mattes RD, Popkin BM. "Nonnutritive Sweetener Consumption in Humans: Effects on Appetite and Food Intake and Their Putative Mechanisms." *American Journal of Clinical Nutrition* 89 (2009): 1–14.

Nettleton JA, Lutsey PL, Wang Y, et al. "Diet Soda Intake and Risk of Incident Metabolic Syndrome and Type 2 Diabetes in the Multi-Ethnic Study of Atherosclerosis (MESA)." *Diabetes Care* 32 (2009): 688–694.

Yang Q. "Gain Weight by 'Going Diet?' Artificial Sweeteners and the Neurobiology of Sugar Cravings: Neuroscience 2010." *Yale Journal of Biology and Medicine* 83 (2010): 101–108.

Juicing Is the Best Way to Get Nutrients

Bazzano LA, Li TY, Joshipura KJ, Hu FB. "Intake of Fruit, Vegetables, and Fruit Juices and Risk of Diabetes in Women." *Diabetes Care* 31 (2008): 1311–1317.

Hurley J, Schmidt S. "All Juiced Up!" *Nutrition Action Healthletter*, July/August 1995, p. 11.

Odegaard AO, Koh WP, Arakawa K, et al. "Soft Drink and Juice Consumption and Risk of Physician-Diagnosed Incident Type 2 Diabetes: The Singapore Chinese Health Study." *American Journal of Epidemiology* 171 (2010): 701–708.

Stanhope KL, Schwarz JM, Keim NL, et al. "Consuming Fructose-Sweetened, Not Glucose-Sweetened, Beverages Increases Visceral Adiposity and Lipids and Decreases Insulin Sensitivity in Overweight/Obese Humans." *Journal of Clinical Investigation* 119 (2009): 1322–1334.

Cranberry Juice Prevents Urinary Infections

Jepson RG, Craig JC. "Cranberries for Preventing Urinary Tract Infections." *Cochrane Database of Systematic Reviews* (2008): CD001321.

Jepson RG, Mihaljevic L, Craig J. "Cranberries for Treating Urinary Tract Infections." *Cochrane Database of Systematic Reviews* (2000): CD001322.

Matsushima M, Suzuki T, Masui A, et al. "Growth Inhibitory Action of Cranberry on *Helicobacter pylori*." *Journal of Gastroenterology and Hepatology* 23 [Suppl 2] (2008): S175–S180.

Sobota AE. "Inhibition of Bacterial Adherence by Cranberry Juice: Potential Use for the Treatment of Urinary Tract Infections." *Journal of Urology* 131 (1984): 1013–1016.

Stothers L. "A Randomized Trial to Evaluate Effectiveness and Cost Effectiveness of Naturopathic Cranberry Products as Prophylaxis against Urinary Tract Infection in Women." *Canadian Journal of Urology* 9 (2002): 1558–1562.

Zhang L, Ma J, Pan K, et al. "Efficacy of Cranberry Juice on *Helicobacter pylori* Infection: A Double-Blind, Randomized Placebo-Controlled Trial." *Helicobacter* 10 (2005): 139–145.

Zikria J, Goldman R, Ansell J. "Cranberry Juice and Warfarin: When Bad Publicity Trumps Science." *American Journal of Medicine* 123 (2010): 384–392.

Green Tea Promotes Weight Loss

Dulloo AG, Duret C, Rohrer D, et al. "Efficacy of a Green Tea Extract Rich in Catechin Polyphenols and Caffeine in Increasing 24-h Energy Expenditure and Fat Oxidation in Humans." *American Journal of Clinical Nutrition* 70 (1999): 1040–1045.

"Look Ten Years Younger in Ten Days," *Oprah Winfrey Show,* November 10, 2004.

Phung OJ, Baker WL, Matthews LJ, et al. "Effect of Green Tea Catechins with or without Caffeine on Anthropometric Measures: A Systematic Review and Meta-Analysis." *American Journal of Clinical Nutrition* 91 (2010): 73–81.

Sarma DN, Barrett ML, Chavez ML, et al. "Safety of Green Tea Extracts: A Systematic Review by the US Pharmacopeia." *Drug Safety* 31 (2008): 469–484.

Westerterp-Plantenga M, Diepvens K, Joosen AM, et al. "Metabolic Effects of Spices, Teas, and Caffeine." *Physiology & Behavior* 89 (2006): 85–91.

Zijp IM, Korver O, Tijburg LB. "Effect of Tea and Other Dietary Factors on Iron Absorption." *Critical Reviews in Food Science and Nutrition* 40 (2000): 371–398.

2. FAT CHANCE

Butter Is More Healthful Than Margarine

Abumweis SS, Barake R, Jones PJ. "Plant Sterols/Stanols as Cholesterol Lowering Agents: A Meta-Analysis of Randomized Controlled Trials." *Food & Nutrition Research* 52 (2008): doi: 10.3402/fnr.v52i0.1811.

Gillman MW, Cupples LA, Gagnon D, et al. "Margarine Intake and Subsequent Coronary Heart Disease in Men." *Epidemiology* 8 (1997): 144–149.

Lichtenstein AH, Ausman LM, Jalbert SM, Schaefer EJ. "Effects of Different Forms of Dietary Hydrogenated Fats on Serum Lipoprotein Cholesterol Levels." *New England Journal of Medicine* 340 (1999): 1933–1940.

Willett WC, Stampfer MJ, Manson JE, et al. "Intake of Trans Fatty Acids and Risk of Coronary Heart Disease among Women." *Lancet* 341 (1993): 581–585.

Olive Is the Most Healthful Type of Vegetable Oil

Astorg P. "Dietary N-6 and N-3 Polyunsaturated Fatty Acids and Prostate Cancer Risk: A Review of Epidemiological and Experimental Evidence." *Cancer Causes & Control* 15 (2004): 367–386.

Covas MI, Nyyssönen K, Poulsen HE, et al. "The Effect of Polyphenols in Olive Oil on Heart Disease Risk Factors: A Randomized Trial." *Annals of Internal Medicine* 145 (2006): 333–341.

Gardner CD, Kraemer HC. "Monounsaturated Versus Polyunsaturated Dietary Fat and Serum Lipids: A Meta-Analysis." *Arteriosclerosis, Thrombosis, and Vascular Biology* 15 (1995): 1917–1927.

Jakobsen MU, O'Reilly EJ, Heitmann BL, et al. "Major Types of Dietary Fat and Risk of Coronary Heart Disease: A Pooled Analysis of 11 Cohort Studies." *American Journal of Clinical Nutrition* 89 (2009): 1425–1432.

Lada AT, Rudel LL. "Dietary Monounsaturated Versus Polyunsaturated Fatty Acids: Which Is Really Better for Protection from Coronary Heart Disease?" *Current Opinion in Lipidology* 14 (2003): 41–46.

Murff HJ, Shu XO, Li H, et al. "Dietary Polyunsaturated Fatty Acids and Breast Cancer Risk in Chinese Women: A Prospective Cohort Study." *International Journal of Cancer* 128 (2011): 1434–1441.

Fish Oil Prevents Heart Disease

Dyerberg J. "Coronary Heart Disease in Greenland Inuit: A Paradox. Implications for Western Diet Patterns." *Arctic Medical Research* 48 (1989): 47–54.

Kris-Etherton PM, Harris WS, Appel LJ, et al. "Fish Consumption, Fish Oil, Omega-3 Fatty Acids, and Cardiovascular Disease." *Circulation* 106 (2002): 2747–2757.

Lavie CJ, Milani RV, Mehra MR, Ventura HO. "Omega-3 Polyunsaturated Fatty Acids and Cardiovascular Diseases." *Journal of the American College of Cardiology* 54 (2009): 585–594.

Marik PE, Varon J. "Omega-3 Dietary Supplements and the Risk of Cardiovascular Events: A Systematic Review." *Clinical Cardiology* 32 (2009): 365–372.

Saito Y, Yokoyama M, Origasa H, et al. "Effects of EPA on Coronary Artery Disease in Hypercholesterolemic Patients with Multiple Risk Factors: Sub-Analysis of

Primary Prevention Cases from the Japan EPA Lipid Intervention Study (JELIS)." *Atherosclerosis* 200 (2008): 135–140.

Ulven SM, Kirkhus B, Lamglait A, et al. "Metabolic Effects of Krill Oil Are Essentially Similar to Those of Fish Oil but at Lower Dose of EPA and DHA, in Healthy Volunteers." *Lipids* 46 (2011): 37–46.

Wang C, Harris WS, Chung M, et al. "N-3 Fatty Acids from Fish or Fish-Oil Supplements, but Not Alpha-Linolenic Acid, Benefit Cardiovascular Disease Outcomes in Primary- and Secondary-Prevention Studies: A Systematic Review." *American Journal of Clinical Nutrition* 84 (2006): 5–17

Eggs Are Bad for Your Heart

Djoussé L, Gaziano JM. "Dietary Cholesterol and Coronary Artery Disease: A Systematic Review." *Current Atherosclerosis Reports* 11 (2009): 418–422.

Djoussé L, Gaziano JM. "Egg Consumption and Risk of Heart Failure in the Physicians' Health Study." *Circulation* 117 (2008): 512–516.

Djoussé L, Gaziano JM. "Egg Consumption in Relation to Cardiovascular Disease and Mortality: The Physicians' Health Study." *American Journal of Clinical Nutrition* 87 (2008): 964–969.

Djoussé L, Gaziano JM, Buring JE, Lee IM. "Egg Consumption and Risk of Type 2 Diabetes in Men and Women." *Diabetes Care* 32 (2009): 295–300.

Fernandez ML. "Dietary Cholesterol Provided by Eggs and Plasma Lipoproteins in Healthy Populations." *Current Opinion in Clinical Nutrition & Metabolic Care* 9 (2006): 8–12.

Houston DK, Ding J, Lee JS, et al. "Dietary Fat and Cholesterol and Risk of Cardiovascular Disease in Older Adults: The Health ABC Study." *Nutrition, Metabolism & Cardiovascular Diseases* 21 (2011): 430–437.

Hu FB, Stampfer MJ, Rimm EB, et al. "A Prospective Study of Egg Consumption and Risk of Cardiovascular Disease in Men and Women." *Journal of the American Medical Association* 281 (1999): 1387–1394.

Nakamura Y, Iso H, Kita Y, et al. "Egg Consumption, Serum Total Cholesterol Concentrations and Coronary Heart Disease Incidence: Japan Public Health Center-Based Prospective Study." *British Journal of Nutrition* 96 (2006): 921–928.

Wallis, C. "Hold the Eggs and Butter; Cholesterol Is Proved Deadly, and Our Diets May Never Be the Same," *Time*, March 26, 1984, p. 56.

Zazpe I, Beunza JJ, Bes-Rastrollo M, et al. "Egg Consumption and Risk of Cardio-vascular Disease in the SUN Project." *European Journal of Clinical Nutrition* 65 (2011): 676–682.

Nuts Prevent Heart Attacks

Fraser GE, Sabaté J, Beeson WL, Strahan TM. "A Possible Protective Effect of Nut Consumption on Risk of Coronary Heart Disease: The Adventist Health Study." *Archives of Internal Medicine* 152 (1992): 1416–1424.

Martínez-González MA, Bes-Rastrollo M. "Nut Consumption, Weight Gain and Obesity: Epidemiological Evidence." *Nutrition, Metabolism & Cardiovascular Diseases* 21 [Suppl 1] (2011): S40–S45.

Sabaté J, Ang Y. "Nuts and Health Outcomes: New Epidemiologic Evidence." *American Journal of Clinical Nutrition* 89 (2009): 1643S–1648S.

Sabaté J, Oda K, Ros E. "Nut Consumption and Blood Lipid Levels: A Pooled Analysis of 25 Intervention Trials." *Archives of Internal Medicine* 170 (2010): 821–827.

Saturated Fat Is Bad for Your Heart

Assunção ML, Ferreira HS, dos Santos AF, et al. "Effects of Dietary Coconut Oil on the Biochemical and Anthropometric Profiles of Women Presenting Abdominal Obesity." *Lipids* 44 (2009): 593–601.

Erkkilä A, de Mello VD, Risérus U, Laaksonen DE. "Dietary Fatty Acids and Cardiovascular Disease: An Epidemiological Approach." *Progress in Lipid Research* 47 (2008): 172–187.

Keys A, Aravanis C, van Buchem FSP, et al. "The Diet and All-Causes Death Rate in the Seven Countries Study." *Lancet* 8237 (1981): 58–61.

Ladeia AM, Costa-Matos E, Barata-Passos R, Costa Guimarães A. "A Palm Oil–Rich Diet May Reduce Serum Lipids in Healthy Young Individuals." *Nutrition* 24 (2008): 11–15.

Micha R, Mozaffarian D. "Saturated Fat and Cardiometabolic Risk Factors, Coronary Heart Disease, Stroke, and Diabetes: A Fresh Look at the Evidence." *Lipids* 45 (2010): 893–905.

Mozaffarian D, Micha R, Wallace S. "Effects on Coronary Heart Disease of Increasing Polyunsaturated Fat in Place of Saturated Fat: A Systematic Review and Meta-Analysis of Randomized Controlled Trials." *PLoS Medicine* 7 (2010): e1000252.

Siri-Tarino PW, Sun Q, Hu FB, Krauss RM. "Meta-Analysis of Prospective Cohort Studies Evaluating the Association of Saturated Fat with Cardiovascular Disease." *American Journal of Clinical Nutrition* 91 (2010): 535–546.

Trans Fats Are Harmful

Mozaffarian D, Aro A, Willett WC. "Health Effects of Trans-Fatty Acids: Experimental and Observational Evidence." *European Journal of Clinical Nutrition* 63 [Suppl 2] (2009): S5–S21.

Mozaffarian D, Katan MB, Ascherio A, et al. "Trans Fatty Acids and Cardiovascular Disease." *New England Journal of Medicine* 354 (2006): 1601–1613.

3. CARB GAMES

Carbs Make You Gain Weight

Foster GD, Wyatt HR, Hill JO, et al. "Weight and Metabolic Outcomes after 2 Years on a Low-Carbohydrate Versus Low-Fat Diet: A Randomized Trial." *Annals of Internal Medicine* 153 (2010): 147–157.

Hession M, Rolland C, Kulkarni U, et al. "Systematic Review of Randomized Controlled Trials of Low-Carbohydrate Vs. Low-Fat/Low-Calorie Diets in the Management of Obesity and Its Comorbidities." *Obesity Reviews* 10 (2009): 36–50.

Sacks FM, Bray GA, Carey VJ, et al. "Comparison of Weight-Loss Diets with Different Compositions of Fat, Protein, and Carbohydrates." *New England Journal of Medicine* 360 (2009): 859–873.

Sichieri R, Moura AS, Genelhu V, et al. "An 18-Month Randomized Trial of a Low-Glycemic-Index Diet and Weight Change in Brazilian Women." *American Journal of Clinical Nutrition* 86 (2007): 707–713.

Van Dam RM, Seidell JC. "Carbohydrate Intake and Obesity." *European Journal of Clinical Nutrition* 61 [Suppl 1] (2007): S75–S99.

Carbs Help You Lose Weight

Bodinham CL, Frost GS, Robertson MD. "Acute Ingestion of Resistant Starch Reduces Food Intake in Healthy Adults." *British Journal of Nutrition* 103 (2010): 917–922.

de Roos N, Heijnen ML, de Graaf C, et al. "Resistant Starch Has Little Effect on Appetite, Food Intake and Insulin Secretion of Healthy Young Men." *European Journal of Clinical Nutrition* 49 (1995): 532–541.

Higgins JA, Higbee DR, Donahoo WT, et al. "Resistant Starch Consumption Promotes Lipid Oxidation." *Nutrition & Metabolism* (London) 1 (2004): 8.

Johnston KL, Thomas EL, Bell JD, et al. "Resistant Starch Improves Insulin Sensitivity in Metabolic Syndrome." *Diabetic Medicine* 27 (2010): 391–397.

Keenan MJ, Zhou J, McCutcheon KL, et al. "Effects of Resistant Starch, a Non-Digestible Fermentable Fiber, on Reducing Body Fat." *Obesity* (Silver Spring) 14 (2006): 1523–1534.

Slavin JL. "Dietary Fiber and Body Weight." *Nutrition* 21 (2005): 411–418.

Willis HJ, Eldridge AL, Beiseigel J, et al. "Greater Satiety Response with Resistant Starch and Corn Bran in Human Subjects." *Nutrition Research* 29 (2009): 100–105.

Multigrain Foods Are Good for You

de Munter JS, Hu FB, Spiegelman D, et al. "Whole Grain, Bran, and Germ Intake and Risk of Type 2 Diabetes: A Prospective Cohort Study and Systematic Review." *PLoS Medicine* 4 (2007): e261.

McIntosh GH, Noakes M, Royle PJ, Foster PR. "Whole-Grain Rye and Wheat Foods and Markers of Bowel Health in Overweight Middle-Aged Men." *American Journal of Clinical Nutrition* 77 (2003): 967–974.

Seal CJ. "Whole Grains and CVD Risk." *Proceedings of the Nutrition Society* 65 (2006): 24–34.

Oats Lower Cholesterol

Kelly SA, Summerbell CD, Brynes A, et al. "Wholegrain Cereals for Coronary Heart Disease." *Cochrane Database of Systematic Reviews* (2007): CD005051.

Kowalski RE. *The 8-Week Cholesterol Cure*. New York: Harper & Row, 1987.

Othman RA, Moghadasian MH, Jones PJ. "Cholesterol-Lowering Effects of Oat β-glucan." *Nutrition Reviews* 69 (2011): 299–309.

Swain JF, Rouse IL, Curley CB, Sacks FM. "Comparison of the Effects of Oat Bran and Low-Fiber Wheat on Serum Lipoprotein Levels and Blood Pressure." *New England Journal of Medicine* 322 (1990): 147–152.

Theuwissen E, Mensink RP. "Water-Soluble Dietary Fibers and Cardiovascular Disease." *Physiology & Behavior* 94 (2008): 285–292.

Gluten Is Harmful

Hasselbeck E. *The G-Free Diet: A Gluten-Free Survival Guide*. New York: Center Street, 2009, p. 11.

Millward C, Ferriter M, Calver S, Connell-Jones G. "Gluten- and Casein-Free Diets for Autistic Spectrum Disorder." *Cochrane Database of Systematic Reviews* (2008): CD003498.

Niewinski MM. "Advances in Celiac Disease and Gluten-Free Diet." *Journal of the American Dietetic Association* 108 (2008): 661–672.

Whiteley P, Haracopos D, Knivsberg AM, et al. "The ScanBrit Randomised, Controlled, Single-Blind Study of a Gluten- and Casein-Free Dietary Intervention for Children with Autism Spectrum Disorders." *Nutritional Neuroscience* 13 (2010): 87–100.

Fiber Prevents Colorectal Cancer

Bonnema AL, Kolberg LW, Thomas W, Slavin JL. "Gastrointestinal Tolerance of Chicory Inulin Products." *Journal of the American Dietetic Association* 110 (2010): 865–868.

Burkitt DP. *Don't Forget Fibre in Your Diet.* London: Martin Dunitz, 1979.

Burkitt DP. "Epidemiology of Cancer of the Colon and Rectum." *Cancer* 28 (1971): 3–13.

de Munter JS, Hu FB, Spiegelman D, et al. "Whole Grain, Bran, and Germ Intake and Risk of Type 2 Diabetes: A Prospective Cohort Study and Systematic Review." *PLoS Medicine* 4 (2007): e261.

Erkkilä AT, Lichtenstein AH. "Fiber and Cardiovascular Disease Risk: How Strong Is the Evidence?" *Journal of Cardiovascular Nursing* 21 (2006): 3–8.

Howe GR, Benito E, Castelleto R, et al. "Dietary Intake of Fiber and Decreased Risk of Cancers of the Colon and Rectum: Evidence from the Combined Analysis of 13 Case-Control Studies." *Journal of the National Cancer Institute* 84 (1992): 1887–1896.

Lanza E, Yu B, Murphy G, et al. "The Polyp Prevention Trial Continued Follow-Up Study: No Effect of a Low-Fat, High-Fiber, High-Fruit-and-Vegetable Diet on Adenoma Recurrence Eight Years after Randomization." *Cancer Epidemiology, Biomarkers & Prevention* 16 (2007): 1745–1752.

Park Y, Hunter DJ, Spiegelman D, et al. "Dietary Fiber Intake and Risk of Colorectal Cancer: A Pooled Analysis of Prospective Cohort Studies." *Journal of the American Medical Association* 294 (2005): 2849–2857.

Park Y, Subar AF, Hollenbeck A, Schatzkin A. "Dietary Fiber Intake and Mortality in the NIH-AARP Diet and Health Study." *Archives of Internal Medicine* 171 (2011): 1061–1068.

Schatzkin A, Lanza E, Corle D, et al. "Lack of Effect of a Low-Fat, High-Fiber Diet on the Recurrence of Colorectal Adenomas. Polyp Prevention Trial Study Group." *New England Journal of Medicine* 342 (2000): 1149–1155.

Schatzkin A, Mouw T, Park Y, et al. "Dietary Fiber and Whole-Grain Consumption in Relation to Colorectal Cancer in the NIH-AARP Diet and Health Study." *American Journal of Clinical Nutrition* 85 (2007): 1353–1360.

4. SUGAR AND SPICE

High-Fructose Corn Syrup Is Worse for You Than Sugar

Bocarsly ME, Powell ES, Avena NM, Hoebel BG. "High-Fructose Corn Syrup Causes Characteristics of Obesity in Rats: Increased Body Weight, Body Fat and Triglyceride Levels." *Pharmacology Biochemistry and Behavior* 97 (2010): 101–106.

Bray GA, Nielsen SJ, Popkin BM. "Consumption of High-Fructose Corn Syrup in Beverages May Play a Role in the Epidemic of Obesity." *American Journal of Clinical Nutrition* 79 (2004): 537–543.

Moeller SM, Fryhofer SA, Osbahr AJ, et al. "The Effects of High Fructose Syrup." *Journal of the American College of Nutrition* 28 (2009): 619–626.

Soenen S, Westerterp-Plantenga MS. "No Differences in Satiety or Energy Intake after High-Fructose Corn Syrup, Sucrose, or Milk Preloads." *American Journal of Clinical Nutrition* 86 (2007): 1586–1594.

Stanhope KL, Griffen SC, Bair BR, et al. "Twenty-Four-Hour Endocrine and Metabolic Profiles Following Consumption of High-Fructose Corn Syrup-, Sucrose-, Fructose-, and Glucose-Sweetened Beverages with Meals." *American Journal of Clinical Nutrition* 87 (2008): 1194–1203.

Stanhope KL, Schwarz JM, Keim NL, et al. "Consuming Fructose-Sweetened, Not Glucose-Sweetened, Beverages Increases Visceral Adiposity and Lipids and Decreases Insulin Sensitivity in Overweight/Obese Humans." *Journal of Clinical Investigation* 119 (2009): 1322–1334.

Tappy L, Lê KA, Tran C, Paquot N. "Fructose and Metabolic Diseases: New Findings, New Questions." *Nutrition* 26 (2010): 1044–1049.

Honey Is More Healthful Than Sugar

Al-Waili NS. "Natural Honey Lowers Plasma Glucose, C-Reactive Protein, Homocysteine, and Blood Lipids in Healthy, Diabetic, and Hyperlipidemic Subjects: Comparison with Dextrose and Sucrose." *Journal of Medicinal Food* 7 (2004): 100–107.

Jull AB, Rodgers A, Walker N. "Honey as a Topical Treatment for Wounds." *Cochrane Database of Systematic Reviews* (2008): CD005083.

Münstedt K, Sheybani B, Hauenschild A, et al. "Effects of Basswood Honey, Honey-Comparable Glucose-Fructose Solution, and Oral Glucose Tolerance Test Solution on Serum Insulin, Glucose, and C-Peptide Concentrations in Healthy Subjects." *Journal of Medicinal Food* 11 (2008): 424–428.

Phillips KM, Carlsen MH, Blomhoff R. "Total Antioxidant Content of Alternatives to Refined Sugar." *Journal of the American Dietetic Association* 109 (2009): 64–71.

Yaghoobi N, Al-Waili N, Ghayour-Mobarhan M, et al. "Natural Honey and Cardiovascular Risk Factors; Effects on Blood Glucose, Cholesterol, Triacylglycerol, CRP, and Body Weight Compared with Sucrose." *ScientificWorldJournal* 8 (2008): 463–469.

Aspartame Is Unsafe

European Commission. "Opinion of the Scientific Committee on Food: Update on the Safety of Aspartame." December 10, 2002. http://ec.europa.eu/food/fs/sc/scf/out155_en.pdf.

Lim U, Subar AF, Mouw T, et al. "Consumption of Aspartame-Containing Beverages and Incidence of Hematopoietic and Brain Malignancies." *Cancer Epidemiology, Biomarkers & Prevention* 15 (2006): 1654–1659.

Magnuson BA, Burdock GA, Doull J, et al. "Aspartame: A Safety Evaluation Based on Current Use Levels, Regulations, and Toxicological and Epidemiological Studies." *Critical Reviews in Toxicology* 37 (2007): 629–727.

Schiffman SS, Buckley CE, Sampson HA, et al. "Aspartame and Susceptibility to Headache." *New England Journal of Medicine* 317 (1987): 1181–1185.

Soffritti M, Belpoggi F, Degli Esposti D, et al. "First Experimental Demonstration of the Multipotential Carcinogenic Effects of Aspartame Administered in the Feed to Sprague-Dawley Rats." *Environmental Health Perspectives* 114 (2006): 379–385.

Soffritti M, Belpoggi F, Manservigi M, et al. "Aspartame Administered in Feed, Beginning Prenatally through Life Span, Induces Cancers of the Liver and Lung in Male Swiss Mice." *American Journal of Industrial Medicine* 53 (2010): 1197–1206.

Van den Eeden SK, Koepsell TD, Longstreth WT Jr., et al. "Aspartame Ingestion and Headaches: A Randomized Crossover Trial." *Neurology* 44 (1994): 1787–1793.

Sea Salt Is More Healthful Than Regular Salt

Institute of Medicine. *Strategies to Reduce Sodium Intake in the United States.* Washington, DC: The National Academies Press, 2010.

MSG Is Harmful

Freeman M. "Reconsidering the Effects of Monosodium Glutamate: A Literature Review." *Journal of the American Academy of Nurse Practitioners* 18 (2006): 482–486.

Jinap S, Hajeb P. "Glutamate: Its Applications in Food and Contribution to Health." *Appetite* 55 (2010): 1–10.

Kwok R. "Chinese Restaurant Syndrome." *New England Journal of Medicine* 278 (1968): 796.

Raiten DJ, Talbot JM, Fisher KD, eds. "Executive Summary from the Report: Analysis of Adverse Reactions to Monosodium Glutamate (MSG)." *Journal of Nutrition* 125 (1995): 2891S–2906S.

Williams AN, Woessner KM. "Monosodium Glutamate 'Allergy': Menace or Myth?" *Clinical & Experimental Allergy* 39 (2009): 640–646.

Cinnamon Is Effective Against Diabetes

Akilen R, Tsiami A, Devendra D, Robinson N. "Glycated Haemoglobin and Blood Pressure–Lowering Effect of Cinnamon in Multi-Ethnic Type 2 Diabetic Patients in the UK: A Randomized, Placebo-Controlled, Double-Blind Clinical Trial." *Diabetic Medicine* 27 (2010): 1159–1167.

Baker WL, Gutierrez-Williams G, White CM, et al. "Effect of Cinnamon on Glucose Control and Lipid Parameters." *Diabetes Care* 31 (2008): 41–43.

Jarvill-Taylor KJ, Anderson RA, Graves DJ. "A Hydroxychalcone Derived from Cinnamon Functions as a Mimetic for Insulin in 3T3-L1 Adipocytes." *Journal of the American College of Nutrition* 20 (2001): 327–336.

Khan A, Safdar M, Ali Khan MM, et al. "Cinnamon Improves Glucose and Lipids of People with Type 2 Diabetes." *Diabetes Care* 26 (2003): 3215–3218.

Kirkham S, Akilen R, Sharma S, Tsiami A. "The Potential of Cinnamon to Reduce Blood Glucose Levels in Patients with Type 2 Diabetes and Insulin Resistance." *Diabetes, Obesity and Metabolism* 11 (2009): 1100–1113.

Pham AQ, Kourlas H, Pham DQ. "Cinnamon Supplementation in Patients with Type 2 Diabetes Mellitus." *Pharmacotherapy* 27 (2007): 595–599.

Zoladz PR, Raudenbush B. "Cognitive Enhancement through Stimulation of the Chemical Senses." *North American Journal of Psychology* 7 (2005): 125–140.

5. DOWN THE GARDEN PATH

Produce Grown Locally Is Most Healthful

Connor AM, Luby JJ, Hancock JF, et al. "Changes in Fruit Antioxidant Activity among Blueberry Cultivars during Cold-Temperature Storage." *Journal of Agricultural and Food Chemistry* 50 (2002): 893–898.

Ferretti G, Bacchetti T, Belleggia A, Neri D. "Cherry Antioxidants: From Farm to Table." *Molecules* 15 (2010): 6993–7005.

Grover J, Goldberg M. "False Claims, Lies Caught on Tape at Farmers Markets." NBC LA, September 23, 2010. www.nbclosangeles.com/news/local/Hidden-Camera-Investigation-Farmers-Markets-103577594.html.

Kalt W, Forney CF, Martin A, Prior RL. "Antioxidant Capacity, Vitamin C, Phenolics, and Anthocyanins after Fresh Storage of Small Fruits." *Journal of Agricultural and Food Chemistry* 47 (1999): 4638–4644.

Kevers C, Falkowski M, Tabart J, et al. "Evolution of Antioxidant Capacity during Storage of Selected Fruits and Vegetables." *Journal of Agricultural and Food Chemistry* 55 (2007): 8596–8603.

Chocolate Is Good for You

Buijsse B, Feskens EJ, Kok FJ, Kromhout D. "Cocoa Intake, Blood Pressure, and Cardiovascular Mortality: The Zutphen Elderly Study." *Archives of Internal Medicine* 166 (2006): 411–417.

Buijsse B, Weikert C, Drogan D, et al. "Chocolate Consumption in Relation to Blood Pressure and Risk of Cardiovascular Disease in German Adults." *European Heart Journal* 31 (2010): 1616–1623.

Ding EL, Hutfless SM, Ding X, Girotra S. "Chocolate and Prevention of Cardio-vascular Disease: A Systematic Review." *Nutrition & Metabolism* (London) 3 (2006): 2.

Huxley RR, Neil HA. "The Relation between Dietary Flavonol Intake and Coronary Heart Disease Mortality: A Meta-Analysis of Prospective Cohort Studies." *European Journal of Clinical Nutrition* 57 (2003): 904–908.

Janszky I, Mukamal KJ, Ljung R, Ahnve S, et al. "Chocolate Consumption and Mortality Following a First Acute Myocardial Infarction: The Stockholm Heart Epidemiology Program." *Journal of Internal Medicine* 266 (2009): 248–257.

Ried K, Sullivan T, Fakler P, et al. "Does Chocolate Reduce Blood Pressure? A Meta-Analysis." *BMC Medicine* 8 (2010): 39.

Tokede OA, Gaziano JM, Djoussé L. "Effects of Cocoa Products/Dark Chocolate on Serum Lipids: A Meta-Analysis." *European Journal of Clinical Nutrition* 65 (2011): 879–886.

Williams S, Tamburic S, Lally C. "Eating Chocolate Can Significantly Protect the Skin from UV Light." *Journal of Cosmetic Dermatology* 8 (2009): 169–173.

Garlic Lowers Cholesterol

Ackermann RT, Mulrow CD, Ramirez G, et al. "Garlic Shows Promise for Improving Some Cardiovascular Risk Factors." *Archives of Internal Medicine* 161 (2001): 813–824.

Alder R, Lookinland S, Berry JA, Williams M. "A Systematic Review of the Effectiveness of Garlic as an Anti-Hyperlipidemic Agent." *Journal of the American Academy of Nurse Practitioners* 15 (2003): 120–129.

Gardner CD, Lawson LD, Block E, et al. "Effect of Raw Garlic vs. Commercial Garlic Supplements on Plasma Lipid Concentrations in Adults with Moderate Hypercholesterolemia: A Randomized Clinical Trial." *Archives of Internal Medicine* 167 (2007): 346–353.

Khoo YS, Aziz Z. "Garlic Supplementation and Serum Cholesterol: A Meta-Analysis." *Journal of Clinical Pharmacy and Therapeutics* 34 (2009): 133–145.

Lissiman E, Bhasale AL, Cohen M. "Garlic for the Common Cold." *Cochrane Database of Systematic Reviews* (2009): CD006206.

Rahman K, Lowe GM. "Garlic and Cardiovascular Disease: A Critical Review." Journal of Nutrition 136 [Suppl 3] (2006): 736S–740S.

Ried K, Frank OR, Stocks NP, et al. "Effect of Garlic on Blood Pressure: A Systematic Review and Meta-Analysis." *BMC Cardiovascular Disorders* 8 (2008): 13.

Raw Veggies Are More Nutritious Than Cooked

Chu M, Seltzer TF. "Myxedema Coma Induced by Ingestion of Raw Bok Choy." *New England Journal of Medicine* 362 (2010): 1945–1946.

Dewanto V, Wu X, Adom KK, Liu RH. "Thermal Processing Enhances the Nutritional Value of Tomatoes by Increasing Total Antioxidant Activity." *Journal of Agricultural and Food Chemistry* 50 (2002): 3010–3014.

Galgano F, Favati F, Caruso M, et al. "The Influence of Processing and Preservation on the Retention of Health-Promoting Compounds in Broccoli." *Journal of Food Science* 72 (2007): S130–S135.

Jiménez-Monreal AM, García-Diz L, Martínez-Tomé M, et al. "Influence of Cooking Methods on Antioxidant Activity of Vegetables." *Journal of Food Science* 74 (2009): H97–H103.

López-Berenguer C, Carvajal M, Moreno DA, García-Viguera C. "Effects of Microwave Cooking Conditions on Bioactive Compounds Present in Broccoli Inflorescences." *Journal of Agricultural and Food Chemistry* 55 (2007): 10001–10007.

Miglio C, Chiavaro E, Visconti A, et al. "Effects of Different Cooking Methods on Nutritional and Physicochemical Characteristics of Selected Vegetables." *Journal of Agricultural and Food Chemistry* 56 (2008): 139–147.

Pellegrini N, Chiavaro E, Gardana C, et al. "Effect of Different Cooking Methods on Color, Phytochemical Concentration, and Antioxidant Capacity of Raw and Frozen Brassica Vegetables." *Journal of Agricultural and Food Chemistry* 58 (2010): 4310–4321.

Organic Produce Is More Healthful Than Conventional Produce

Bouchard MF, Bellinger DC, Wright RO, Weisskopf MG. "Attention-Deficit/Hyperactivity Disorder and Urinary Metabolites of Organophosphate Pesticides." *Pediatrics* 125 (2010): e1270–e1277.

Colosio C, Tiramani M, Brambilla G, et al. "Neurobehavioural Effects of Pesticides with Special Focus on Organophosphorus Compounds: Which Is the Real Size of the Problem? *Neurotoxicology* 30 (2009): 1155–1161.

Dangour AD, Dodhia SK, Hayter A, et al. "Nutritional Quality of Organic Foods: A Systematic Review." *American Journal of Clinical Nutrition* 90 (2009): 680–685.

Eskenazi B, Rosas LG, Marks AR, et al. "Pesticide Toxicity and the Developing Brain." *Basic & Clinical Pharmacology & Toxicology* 102 (2008): 228–236.

"Large Majorities See Organic Food As Safer, Better for the Environment and Healthier—but Also More Expensive." The Harris Poll #97, October 8, 2007. www.harrisinteractive.com/vault/Harris-Interactive-Poll-Research-Organic-Food-2007-10.pdf.

Lee JW, Shimizu M, Wansink B. "You Taste What You See: Organic Labels Favorably Bias Taste Perceptions." *Journal of the Federation of American Societies for Experimental Biology* 25 (2011): 610.2.

Magkos F, Arvaniti F, Zampelas A. "Organic Food: Buying More Safety or Just Peace of Mind? A Critical Review of the Literature." *Critical Reviews in Food Science and Nutrition* 46 (2006): 23–56.

Rosas LG, Eskenazi B. "Pesticides and Child Neurodevelopment." *Current Opinion in Pediatrics* 20 (2008): 191–197.

Acai Berries Help You Lose Weight

Adhami VM, Khan N, Mukhtar H. "Cancer Chemoprevention by Pomegranate: Laboratory and Clinical Evidence." *Nutrition and Cancer* 61 (2009): 811–815.

Mertens-Talcott SU, Rios J, Jilma-Stohlawetz P, et al. "Pharmacokinetics of Anthocyanins and Antioxidant Effects after the Consumption of Anthocyanin-Rich Acai Juice and Pulp (*Euterpe oleracea* Mart.) in Human Healthy Volunteers." *Journal of Agricultural and Food Chemistry* 56 (2008): 7796–7802.

Seeram NP, Aviram M, Zhang Y, et al. "Comparison of Antioxidant Potency of Commonly Consumed Polyphenol-Rich Beverages in the United States." *Journal of Agricultural and Food Chemistry* 56 (2008): 1415–1422.

Stowe CB. "The Effects of Pomegranate Juice Consumption on Blood Pressure and Cardiovascular Health." *Complementary Therapies in Clinical Practice* 17 (2011): 113–115.

Soy Wards Off Cancer

Ginsberg B, Milken M. *The Taste for Living Cookbook: Mike Milken's Favorite Recipes for Fighting Cancer.* Santa Monica, CA: CaP CURE, 1998.

Korde LA, Wu AH, Fears T, et al. "Childhood Soy Intake and Breast Cancer Risk in Asian American Women." *Cancer Epidemiology, Biomarkers & Prevention* 18 (2009): 1050–1059.

Nagata C. "Factors to Consider in the Association between Soy Isoflavone Intake and Breast Cancer Risk." *Journal of Epidemiology* 20 (2010): 83–89.

Sathyapalan T, Manuchehri AM, Thatcher NJ, et al. "The Effect of Soy Phytoestrogen Supplementation on Thyroid Status and Cardiovascular Risk Markers in Patients with Subclinical Hypothyroidism: A Randomized, Double-Blind, Crossover Study." *Journal of Clinical Endocrinology & Metabolism* 96 (2011): 1442–1449.

Shu XO, Zheng Y, Cai H, et al. "Soy Food Intake and Breast Cancer Survival." *Journal of the American Medical Association* 302 (2009): 2437–2443.

Trock BJ, Hilakivi-Clarke L, Clarke R. "Meta-Analysis of Soy Intake and Breast Cancer Risk." *Journal of the National Cancer Institute* 98 (2006): 459–471.

Wu AH, Yu MC, Tseng CC, Pike MC. "Epidemiology of Soy Exposures and Breast Cancer Risk." *British Journal of Cancer* 98 (2008): 9–14.

Yan L, Spitznagel EL. "Soy Consumption and Prostate Cancer Risk in Men: A Revisit of a Meta-Analysis." *American Journal of Clinical Nutrition* 89 (2009): 1155–1163.

Tomatoes Prevent Prostate Cancer

Giovannucci E. "Tomatoes, Tomato-Based Products, Lycopene, and Cancer: Review of the Epidemiologic Literature." *Journal of the National Cancer Institute* 91 (1999): 317–331.

Giovannucci E, Rimm EB, Liu Y, et al. "A Prospective Study of Tomato Products, Lycopene, and Prostate Cancer Risk." *Journal of the National Cancer Institute* 94 (2002): 391–398.

Kavanaugh CJ, Trumbo PR, Ellwood KC. "The U.S. Food and Drug Administration's Evidence-Based Review for Qualified Health Claims: Tomatoes, Lycopene, and Cancer." *Journal of the National Cancer Institute* 99 (2007): 1074–1085.

Kirsh VA, Mayne ST, Peters U, et al. "A Prospective Study of Lycopene and Tomato Product Intake and Risk of Prostate Cancer." *Cancer Epidemiology, Biomarkers & Prevention* 15 (2006): 92–98.

Perkins-Veazie P, Collins JK. "Carotenoid Changes of Intact Watermelons after Storage." *Journal of Agricultural and Food Chemistry* 54 (2006): 5868–5874.

6. MEATY OR FISHY?

Red Meat Is Bad for You

Bernstein AM, Sun Q, Hu FB, et al. "Major Dietary Protein Sources and Risk of Coronary Heart Disease in Women." *Circulation* 122 (2010): 876–883.

Cross AJ, Ferrucci LM, Risch A, et al. "A Large Prospective Study of Meat Consumption and Colorectal Cancer Risk: An Investigation of Potential Mechanisms Underlying This Association." *Cancer Research* 70 (2010): 2406–2414.

Cross AJ, Leitzmann MF, Gail MH, et al. "A Prospective Study of Red and Processed Meat Intake in Relation to Cancer Risk." *PLoS Medicine* 4 (2007): e325.

Freedman ND, Cross AJ, McGlynn KA, et al. "Association of Meat and Fat Intake with Liver Disease and Hepatocellular Carcinoma in the NIH-AARP Cohort." *Journal of the National Cancer Institute* 102 (2010): 1354–1365.

Larsson SC, Wolk A. "Meat Consumption and Risk of Colorectal Cancer: A Meta-Analysis of Prospective Studies." *International Journal of Cancer* 119 (2006): 2657–2664.

Micha R, Wallace SK, Mozaffarian D. "Red and Processed Meat Consumption and Risk of Incident Coronary Heart Disease, Stroke, and Diabetes Mellitus: A Systematic Review and Meta-Analysis." *Circulation* 121 (2010): 2271–2283.

Norat T, Bingham S, Ferrari P, et al. "Meat, Fish, and Colorectal Cancer Risk: The European Prospective Investigation into Cancer and Nutrition." *Journal of the National Cancer Institute* 97 (2005): 906–916.

Sinha R, Cross AJ, Graubard BI, et al. "Meat Intake and Mortality: A Prospective Study of Over Half a Million People." *Archives of Internal Medicine* 169 (2009): 562–571.

Grass-Fed Beef Is More Healthful Than Grain-Fed Beef

Bhattacharya A, Banu J, Rahman M, et al. "Biological Effects of Conjugated Linoleic Acids in Health and Disease." *Journal of Nutritional Biochemistry* 17 (2006): 789–810.

Daley CA, Abbott A, Doyle PS, et al. "A Review of Fatty Acid Profiles and Antioxidant Content in Grass-Fed and Grain-Fed Beef." *Nutrition Journal* 9 (2010): 10.

Diez-Gonzalez F, Callaway TR, Kizoulis MG, Russell JB. "Grain Feeding and the Dissemination of Acid-Resistant *Escherichia coli* from Cattle." *Science* 281 (1998): 1666–1668.

Leheska JM, Thompson LD, Howe JC, et al. "Effects of Conventional and Grass-Feeding Systems on the Nutrient Composition of Beef." *Journal of Animal Science* 86 (2008): 3575–3585.

McAfee AJ, McSorley EM, Cuskelly GJ, et al. "Red Meat from Animals Offered a Grass Diet Increases Plasma and Platelet N-3 PUFA in Healthy Consumers." *British Journal of Nutrition* 105 (2011): 80–89.

Wang C, Harris WS, Chung M, et al. "N-3 Fatty Acids from Fish or Fish-Oil Supplements, but Not Alpha-Linolenic Acid, Benefit Cardiovascular Disease Outcomes in Primary- and Secondary-Prevention Studies: A Systematic Review." *American Journal of Clinical Nutrition* 84 (2006): 5–17.

World Health Organization. "Joint FAO/OIE/WHO Expert Workshop on Non-Human Antimicrobial Usage and Antimicrobial Resistance: Scientific Assessment." December 2003. www.who.int/foodsafety/publications/micro/en/amr.pdf.

Zhang J, Wall SK, Xu L, Ebner PD. "Contamination Rates and Antimicrobial Resistance in Bacteria Isolated from 'Grass-Fed' Labeled Beef Products." *Foodborne Pathogens and Disease* 7 (2010): 1331–1336.

Well-Done Meat Causes Cancer

Cross AJ, Peters U, Kirsh VA, et al. "A Prospective Study of Meat and Meat Mutagens and Prostate Cancer Risk." *Cancer Research* 65 (2005): 11779–11784.

Knize MG, Sinha R, Rothman N, et al. "Heterocyclic Amine Content in Fast-Food Meat Products." *Food and Chemical Toxicology* 33 (1995): 545–551

Stolzenberg-Solomon RZ, Cross AJ, Silverman DT, et al. "Meat and Meat-Mutagen Intake and Pancreatic Cancer Risk in the NIH-AARP Cohort." *Cancer Epidemiology, Biomarkers & Prevention* 16 (2007): 2664–2675.

Zheng W, Lee SA. "Well-Done Meat Intake, Heterocyclic Amine Exposure, and Cancer Risk." *Nutrition and Cancer* 61 (2009): 437–446.

Kosher Meat Is More Wholesome Than Conventional Meat

Mintel Oxygen Reports. "3 in 5 Kosher Food Buyers Purchase for Food Quality, Not Religion." February 2009. www.mintel.com/press-centre/press-releases/321/3-in-5-kosher-food-buyers-purchase-for-food-quality-not-religion.

Nou X, Delgado J, Patel J, et al. "Prevalence of *Salmonella, Campylobacter* and *Listeria* on Retail Organic and Kosher Poultry Products." *International Association for*

Food Protection Program and Abstract Book, 2007, p. 157. www.ars.usda.gov/research/publications/publications.htm?seq_no_115=207351.

Oscar TP. "Persistence of Salmonella Serotypes on Chicken Skin after Exposure to Kosher Salt and Rinsing." *Journal of Food Safety* 28 (2008): 389–399.

Farmed Salmon Is Less Healthful Than Wild-Caught Salmon

Bayen S, Barlow P, Lee HK, Obbard JP. "Effect of Cooking on the Loss of Persistent Organic Pollutants from Salmon." *Journal of Toxicology and Environmental Health. Part A* 68 (2005): 253–265.

Foran JA, Carpenter DO, Hamilton MC, et al. "Risk-Based Consumption Advice for Farmed Atlantic and Wild Pacific Salmon Contaminated with Dioxins and Dioxin-Like Compounds." *Environmental Health Perspectives* 113 (2005): 552–556.

Hites RA, Foran JA, Carpenter DO, et al. "Global Assessment of Organic Contaminants in Farmed Salmon." *Science* 303 (2004): 226–229.

Kelly BC, Ikonomou MG, Higgs DA, et al. "Mercury and Other Trace Elements in Farmed and Wild Salmon from British Columbia, Canada." *Environmental Toxicology and Chemistry* 27 (2008): 1361–1370.

Mozaffarian D, Rimm EB. "Fish Intake, Contaminants, and Human Health: Evaluating the Risks and the Benefits." *Journal of the American Medical Association* 296 (2006): 1885–1899.

Mercury in Sushi Is Toxic

Auger N, Kofman O, Kosatsky T, Armstrong B. "Low-Level Methylmercury Exposure as a Risk Factor for Neurologic Abnormalities in Adults." *Neurotoxicology* 26 (2005): 149–157.

Burros M. "High Mercury Levels Are Found in Tuna Sushi." *New York Times*, January 23, 2008.

Cox C, Marsh D, Myers G, Clarkson T. "Analysis of Data on Delayed Development from the 1971–72 Outbreak of Methylmercury Poisoning in Iraq: Assessment of Influential Points." *Neurotoxicology* 16 (1995): 727–730.

Debes F, Budtz-Jørgensen E, Weihe P, et al. "Impact of Prenatal Methylmercury Exposure on Neurobehavioral Function at Age 14 Years." *Neurotoxicology and Teratology* 28 (2006): 363–375.

Ekino S, Susa M, Ninomiya T, et al. "Minamata Disease Revisited: An Update on the Acute and Chronic Manifestations of Methyl Mercury Poisoning." *Journal of the Neurological Sciences* 262 (2007): 131–144.

Fortini A. "Jeremy Piven's Fishy Excuse." *Daily Beast*, January 15, 2009.

Hibbeln JR, Davis JM, Steer C, et al. "Maternal Seafood Consumption in Pregnancy and Neurodevelopmental Outcomes in Childhood (ALSPAC Study): An Observational Cohort Study." *Lancet* 369 (2007): 578–585.

"Hold the Mercury: How to Avoid Mercury When Buying Fish." Washington, DC: Oceana, January 1, 2008.

Mozaffarian D, Rimm EB. "Fish Intake, Contaminants, and Human Health: Evaluating the Risks and the Benefits." *Journal of the American Medical Association* 296 (2006): 1885–1899.

Myers GJ, Thurston SW, Pearson AT, et al. "Postnatal Exposure to Methyl Mercury from Fish Consumption: A Review and New Data from the Seychelles Child Development Study." *Neurotoxicology* 30 (2009): 338–349.

Oken E, Radesky JS, Wright RO, et al. "Maternal Fish Intake during Pregnancy, Blood Mercury Levels, and Child Cognition at Age 3 Years in a US Cohort." *American Journal of Epidemiology* 167 (2008): 1171–1181.

Riedel M, Fagen C. "Piven's Fish Tale Begins to Stink." *New York Post,* December 19, 2008.

Stern AH. "A Review of the Studies of the Cardiovascular Health Effects of Methylmercury with Consideration of Their Suitability for Risk Assessment." *Environmental Research* 98 (2005): 133–142.

Weil M, Bressler J, Parsons P, et al. "Blood Mercury Levels and Neurobehavioral Function." *Journal of the American Medical Association* 293 (2005): 1875–1882.

7. MILKING THE SCIENCE

Yogurt Improves Digestion

Chmielewska A, Szajewska H. "Systematic Review of Randomised Controlled Trials: Probiotics for Functional Constipation." *World Journal of Gastroenterology* 16 (2010): 69–75.

Floch MH, Walker WA, Guandalini S, et al. "Recommendations for Probiotic Use—2008." *Journal of Clinical Gastroenterology* 42 [Suppl 2] (2008): S104–S108.

Moayyedi P, Ford AC, Talley NJ, et al. "The Efficacy of Probiotics in the Treatment of Irritable Bowel Syndrome: A Systematic Review." *Gut* 59 (2010): 325–332.

Williams NT. "Probiotics." *American Journal of Health-System Pharmacy* 67 (2010): 449–458.

Yang YX, He M, Hu G, et al. "Effect of a Fermented Milk Containing *Bifidobacterium lactis* DN-173010 on Chinese Constipated Women." *World Journal of Gastroenterology* 14 (2008): 6237–6243.

Raw Milk Is Better for You Than Pasteurized Milk

Basnet S, Schneider M, Gazit A, et al. "Fresh Goat's Milk for Infants: Myths and Realities—A Review." *Pediatrics* 125 (2010): e973–e977.

Centers for Disease Control and Prevention. "Raw Milk Questions and Answers." www.cdc.gov/foodsafety/rawmilk/raw-milk-questions-and-answers.html #risks.

Guh A, Phan Q, Nelson R, et al. "Outbreak of *Escherichia coli* O157 Associated with Raw Milk, Connecticut, 2008." *Clinical Infectious Diseases* 51 (2010): 1411–1417.

Lejeune JT, Rajala-Schultz PJ. "Food Safety: Unpasteurized Milk: A Continued Public Health Threat." *Clinical Infectious Diseases* 48 (2009): 93–100.

Oliver SP, Boor KJ, Murphy SC, Murinda SE. "Food Safety Hazards Associated with Consumption of Raw Milk." *Foodborne Pathogens and Disease* 6 (2009): 793–806.

Riedler J, Braun-Fahrländer C, Eder W, et al. "Exposure to Farming in Early Life and Development of Asthma and Allergy: A Cross-Sectional Survey." *Lancet* 358 (2001): 1129–1133.

Waser M, Michels KB, Bieli C, et al. "Inverse Association of Farm Milk Consumption with Asthma and Allergy in Rural and Suburban Populations across Europe." *Clinical & Experimental Allergy* 37 (2007): 661–670.

Soy Milk Is More Healthful Than Cow's Milk

Gardner CD, Messina M, Kiazand A, et al. "Effect of Two Types of Soy Milk and Dairy Milk on Plasma Lipids in Hypercholesterolemic Adults: A Randomized Trial." *Journal of the American College of Nutrition* 26 (2007): 669–677.

Liu J, Ho SC, Su YX, et al. "Effect of Long-Term Intervention of Soy Isoflavones on Bone Mineral Density in Women: A Meta-Analysis of Randomized Controlled Trials." *Bone* 44 (2009): 948–953.

Soroko S, Holbrook TL, Edelstein S, Barrett-Connor E. "Lifetime Milk Consumption and Bone Mineral Density in Older Women." *American Journal of Public Health* 84 (1994): 1319–1322.

Taku K, Melby MK, Takebayashi J, et al. "Effect of Soy Isoflavone Extract Supplements on Bone Mineral Density in Menopausal Women: Meta-Analysis of Randomized Controlled Trials." *Asia Pacific Journal of Clinical Nutrition* 19 (2010): 33–42.

Taku K, Umegaki K, Sato Y, et al. "Soy Isoflavones Lower Serum Total and LDL Cholesterol in Humans: A Meta-Analysis of 11 Randomized Controlled Trials." *American Journal of Clinical Nutrition* 85 (2007): 1148–1156.

Zhao Y, Martin BR, Weaver CM. "Calcium Bioavailability of Calcium Carbonate Fortified Soymilk Is Equivalent to Cow's Milk in Young Women." *Journal of Nutrition* 135 (2005): 2379–2382.

Milk Is Necessary for Strong Bones

Bischoff-Ferrari HA, Dawson-Hughes B, Baron JA, et al. "Milk Intake and Risk of Hip Fracture in Men and Women: A Meta-Analysis of Prospective Cohort Studies." *Journal of Bone and Mineral Research* 26 (2011): 833–839.

Bischoff-Ferrari HA, Willett WC, Wong JB, et al. "Prevention of Nonvertebral Fractures with Oral Vitamin D and Dose Dependency: A Meta-Analysis of Randomized Controlled Trials." *Archives of Internal Medicine* 169 (2009): 551–561.

Darling AL, Millward DJ, Torgerson DJ, et al. "Dietary Protein and Bone Health: A Systematic Review and Meta-Analysis." *American Journal of Clinical Nutrition* 90 (2009): 1674–1692.

Feskanich D, Willett WC, Colditz GA. "Calcium, Vitamin D, Milk Consumption, and Hip Fractures: A Prospective Study Among Postmenopausal Women." *American Journal of Clinical Nutrition* 77 (2003): 504–511.

Hegsted DM. "Fractures, Calcium, and the Modern Diet." *American Journal of Clinical Nutrition* 74 (2001): 571–573.

Weinsier RL, Krumdieck CL. "Dairy Foods and Bone Health: Examination of the Evidence." *American Journal of Clinical Nutrition* 72 (2000): 681–689.

Dairy Products Cause Cancer

Ahn J, Albanes D, Peters U, et al. "Dairy Products, Calcium Intake, and Risk of Prostate Cancer in the Prostate, Lung, Colorectal, and Ovarian Cancer Screening Trial." *Cancer Epidemiology, Biomarkers & Prevention* 16 (2007): 2623–2630.

"Bovine Somatotropin and the Safety of Cows' Milk: National Institutes of Health Technology Assessment Conference Statement." *Nutrition Reviews* 49 (1991): 227–232.

Cho E, Smith-Warner SA, Spiegelman D, et al. "Dairy Foods, Calcium, and Colorectal Cancer: A Pooled Analysis of 10 Cohort Studies." *Journal of the National Cancer Institute* 96 (2004): 1015–1022.

Gao X, LaValley MP, Tucker KL. "Prospective Studies of Dairy Product and Calcium Intakes and Prostate Cancer Risk: A Meta-Analysis." *Journal of the National Cancer Institute* 97 (2005): 1768–1777.

Genkinger JM, Hunter DJ, Spiegelman D, et al. "Dairy Products and Ovarian Cancer: A Pooled Analysis of 12 Cohort Studies." *Cancer Epidemiology, Biomarkers & Prevention* 15 (2006): 364–372.

Giovannucci E, Rimm EB, Wolk A, et al. "Calcium and Fructose Intake in Relation to Risk of Prostate Cancer." *Cancer Research* 58 (1998): 442–447.

Givens D, Morgan R, Elwood P. "Relationship between Milk Consumption and Prostate Cancer: A Short Review." *Nutrition Bulletin* 33 (2008): 279–286.

Larsson SC, Orsini N, Wolk A. "Milk, Milk Products and Lactose Intake and Ovarian Cancer Risk: A Meta-Analysis of Epidemiological Studies." *International Journal of Cancer* 118 (2006): 431–441.

Michels KB, Mohllajee AP, Roset-Bahmanyar E, et al. "Diet and Breast Cancer: A Review of the Prospective Observational Studies." *Cancer* 109 [Suppl 12] (2007): 2712–2749.

Park SY, Murphy SP, Wilkens LR, et al. "Calcium, Vitamin D, and Dairy Product Intake and Prostate Cancer Risk: The Multiethnic Cohort Study." *American Journal of Epidemiology* 166 (2007): 1259–1269.

Park Y, Mitrou PN, Kipnis V, et al. "Calcium, Dairy Foods, and Risk of Incident and Fatal Prostate Cancer: The NIH-AARP Diet and Health Study." *American Journal of Epidemiology* 166 (2007): 1270–1279.

Dairy Products Promote Weight Loss

Barba G, Russo P. "Dairy Foods, Dietary Calcium and Obesity: A Short Review of the Evidence." *Nutrition, Metabolism & Cardiovascular Diseases* 16 (2006): 445–451.

Huang TT, McCrory MA. "Dairy Intake, Obesity, and Metabolic Health in Children and Adolescents: Knowledge and Gaps." *Nutrition Reviews* 63 (2005): 71–80.

Lanou AJ, Barnard ND. "Dairy and Weight Loss Hypothesis: An Evaluation of the Clinical Trials." *Nutrition Reviews* 66 (2008): 272–279.

Parnes LB. Federal Trade Commission letter to Dr. Neal Barnard, May 3, 2007. www.pcrm.org/news/downloads/FTCResponsetoPCRM.pdf.

Ralston RA, Lee JH, Truby H, et al. "A Systematic Review and Meta-Analysis of Elevated Blood Pressure and Consumption of Dairy Foods." *Journal of Human Hypertension* (2011) February 10 [epub].

Schardt D. "Milking the Data." *Nutrition Action Healthletter*, September 2005, pp. 9–11.

Tong X, Dong JY, Wu ZW, et al. "Dairy Consumption and Risk of Type 2 Diabetes Mellitus: A Meta-Analysis of Cohort Studies." *European Journal of Clinical Nutrition* 65 (2011): 1027–1031.

Trowman R, Dumville JC, Hahn S, Torgerson DJ. "A Systematic Review of the Effects of Calcium Supplementation on Body Weight." *British Journal of Nutrition* 95 (2006): 1033–1038.

Zemel MB, Richards J, Mathis S, et al. "Dairy Augmentation of Total and Central Fat Loss in Obese Subjects." *International Journal of Obesity* (London) 29 (2005): 391–397.

Zemel MB, Richards J, Milstead A, Campbell P. "Effects of Calcium and Dairy on Body Composition and Weight Loss in African-American Adults." *Obesity Research* 13 (2005): 1218–1225.

Zemel MB, Thompson W, Milstead A, et al. "Calcium and Dairy Acceleration of Weight and Fat Loss during Energy Restriction in Obese Adults." *Obesity Research* 12 (2004): 582–590.

8. TAKE (OR LEAVE) YOUR VITAMINS

Vitamin C Fights Colds

Douglas RM, Hemilä H, Chalker E, Treacy B. "Vitamin C for Preventing and Treating the Common Cold." *Cochrane Database of Systematic Reviews* (2007): CD000980.

Heimer KA, Hart AM, Martin LG, Rubio-Wallace S. "Examining the Evidence for the Use of Vitamin C in the Prophylaxis and Treatment of the Common Cold." *Journal of the American Academy of Nurse Practitioners* 21 (2009): 295–300.

Singh M, Das RR. "Zinc for the Common Cold." *Cochrane Database of Systematic Reviews* (2011): CD001364.

Most of Us Need More Vitamin D

Autier P, Gandini S. "Vitamin D Supplementation and Total Mortality: A Meta-Analysis of Randomized Controlled Trials." *Archives of Internal Medicine* 167 (2007): 1730–1737.

Binkley N, Gemar D, Engelke J, et al. "Evaluation of Ergocalciferol or Cholecalciferol Dosing, 1,600 IU Daily or 50,000 IU Monthly in Older Adults." *Journal of Clinical Endocrinology and Metabolism* 96 (2011): 981–988.

Bischoff-Ferrari HA, Dawson-Hughes B, Staehelin HB, et al. "Fall Prevention with Supplemental and Active Forms of Vitamin D: A Meta-Analysis of Randomised Controlled Trials." *BMJ* 339 (2009): b3692.

Bischoff-Ferrari HA, Willett WC, Wong JB, et al. "Prevention of Nonvertebral Fractures with Oral Vitamin D and Dose Dependency: A Meta-Analysis of Randomized Controlled Trials." *Archives of Internal Medicine* 169 (2009): 551–561.

Chung M, Balk EM, Brendel M, et al. *Vitamin D and Calcium: A Systematic Review of Health Outcomes.* Rockville, MD: Agency for Healthcare Research and Quality, 2009.

Eliassen AH, Spiegelman D, Hollis BW, et al. "Plasma 25-Hydroxyvitamin D and Risk of Breast Cancer in the Nurses' Health Study II." *Breast Cancer Research* 13 (2011): R50.

Gandini S, Boniol M, Haukka J, et al. "Meta-Analysis of Observational Studies of Serum 25-Hydroxyvitamin D Levels and Colorectal, Breast and Prostate Cancer and Colorectal Adenoma." *International Journal of Cancer* 128 (2011): 1414–1424.

Heaney RP, Recker RR, Grote J, et al. "Vitamin D(3) Is More Potent Than Vitamin D(2) in Humans." *Journal of Clinical Endocrinology & Metabolism* 96 (2011): E447–E452.

Helzlsouer KJ, VDPP Steering Committee. "Overview of the Cohort Consortium Vitamin D Pooling Project of Rarer Cancers." *American Journal of Epidemiology* 172 (2010): 4–9.

Institute of Medicine. *Dietary Reference Intakes for Calcium and Vitamin D.* Washington, DC: National Academies Press, 2011.

Kolata G. "Report Questions Need for 2 Diet Supplements." *New York Times*, November 29, 2010.

Lappe JM, Travers-Gustafson D, Davies KM, et al. "Vitamin D and Calcium Supplementation Reduces Cancer Risk: Results of a Randomized Trial." *American Journal of Clinical Nutrition* 85 (2007): 1586–1591.

Munger KL, Levin LI, Hollis BW, et al. "Serum 25-Hydroxyvitamin D Levels and Risk of Multiple Sclerosis." *Journal of the American Medical Association* 296 (2006): 2832–2838.

Pittas AG, Chung M, Trikalinos T, et al. "Systematic Review: Vitamin D and Cardiometabolic Outcomes." *Annals of Internal Medicine* 152 (2010): 307–314.

Trivedi DP, Doll R, Khaw KT. "Effect of Four Monthly Oral Vitamin D_3 (cholecalciferol) Supplementation on Fractures and Mortality in Men and Women Living in the Community: Randomised Double Blind Controlled Trial." *BMJ* 326 (2003): 469.

Tuohimaa P, Tenkanen L, Ahonen M, et al. "Both High and Low Levels of Blood Vitamin D Are Associated with a Higher Prostate Cancer Risk: A Longitudinal, Nested Case-Control Study in the Nordic Countries." *International Journal of Cancer* 108 (2004): 104–108.

Wang L, Manson JE, Song Y, Sesso HD. "Systematic Review: Vitamin D and Calcium Supplementation in Prevention of Cardiovascular Events." *Annals of Internal Medicine* 152 (2010): 315–323.

B Vitamins Give You Energy

Balk EM, Raman G, Tatsioni A, et al. "Vitamin B_6, B_{12}, and Folic Acid Supplementation and Cognitive Function: A Systematic Review of Randomized Trials." *Archives of Internal Medicine* 167 (2007): 21–30.

Heckman M, Sherry K, de Mejia, EG. "Energy Drinks: An Assessment of Their Market Size, Consumer Demographics, Ingredient Profile, Functionality, and Regulations in the United States." *Comprehensive Reviews in Food Science and Food Safety* 9 (2010): 303–317.

House AA, Eliasziw M, Cattran DC, et al. "Effect of B-Vitamin Therapy on Progression of Diabetic Nephropathy: A Randomized Controlled Trial." *Journal of the American Medical Association* 303 (2010): 1603–1609.

Lukaski HC. "Vitamin and Mineral Status: Effects on Physical Performance." *Nutrition* 20 (2004): 632–644.

Kaminer Y. "Problematic Use of Energy Drinks by Adolescents." *Child and Adolescent Psychiatric Clinics of North America* 19 (2010): 643–650.

Niacin Improves Cholesterol Levels

Centers for Disease Control and Prevention (CDC). "Use of Niacin in Attempts to Defeat Urine Drug Testing—Five States, January–September 2006." *Morbidity and Mortality Weekly Report* 56 (2007): 365–366.

Duggal JK, Singh M, Attri N, et al. "Effect of Niacin Therapy on Cardiovascular Outcomes in Patients with Coronary Artery Disease." *Journal of Cardiovascular Pharmacology and Therapeutics* 15 (2010): 158–166.

Gibbons LW, Gonzalez V, Gordon N, Grundy S. "The Prevalence of Side Effects with Regular and Sustained-Release Nicotinic Acid." *American Journal of Medicine* 99 (1995): 378–385.

Martí-Carvajal AJ, Solà I, Lathyris D, Salanti G. "Homocysteine Lowering Interventions for Preventing Cardiovascular Events." *Cochrane Database of Systematic Reviews* (2009): CD006612.

Meyers CD, Carr MC, Park S, Brunzell JD. "Varying Cost and Free Nicotinic Acid Content in Over-the-Counter Niacin Preparations for Dyslipidemia." *Annals of Internal Medicine* 139 (2003): 996–1002.

Mittal MK, Florin T, Perrone J, et al. "Toxicity from the Use of Niacin to Beat Urine Drug Screening." *Annals of Emergency Medicine* 50 (2007): 587–590.

National Institutes of Health. "NIH Stops Clinical Trial on Combination Cholesterol Treatment." Press release, May 26, 2011. www.nih.gov/news/health/may2011/nhlbi-26.htm.

Antioxidants Are Good for Your Eyes

Age-Related Eye Disease Study Research Group. "A Randomized, Placebo-Controlled, Clinical Trial of High-Dose Supplementation with Vitamins C and E and Beta Carotene for Age-Related Cataract and Vision Loss: AREDS Report No. 9." *Archives of Ophthalmology* 119 (2001): 1439–1452.

Age-Related Eye Disease Study Research Group. "A Randomized, Placebo-Controlled, Clinical Trial of High-Dose Supplementation with Vitamins C and E, Beta Carotene, and Zinc for Age-Related Macular Degeneration and Vision Loss: AREDS Report No. 8." *Archives of Ophthalmology* 119 (2001): 1417–1436.

Bjelakovic G, Nikolova D, Gluud LL, et al. "Mortality in Randomized Trials of Antioxidant Supplements for Primary and Secondary Prevention: Systematic

Review and Meta-Analysis." *Journal of the American Medical Association* 297 (2007): 842–857.

Chiu CJ, Taylor A. "Nutritional Antioxidants and Age-Related Cataract and Maculopathy." *Experimental Eye Research* 84 (2007): 229–245.

Christen WG, Liu S, Glynn RJ, et al. "Dietary Carotenoids, Vitamins C and E, and Risk of Cataract in Women: A Prospective Study." *Archives of Ophthalmology* 126 (2008): 102–109.

Ma L, Lin XM. "Effects of Lutein and Zeaxanthin on Aspects of Eye Health." *Journal of the Science of Food and Agriculture* 90 (2010): 2–12.

Saremi A, Arora R. "Vitamin E and Cardiovascular Disease." *American Journal of Therapeutics* 17 (2010): e56–e65.

Tan AG, Mitchell P, Flood VM, et al. "Antioxidant Nutrient Intake and the Long-Term Incidence of Age-Related Cataract: The Blue Mountains Eye Study." *American Journal of Clinical Nutrition* 87 (2008): 1899–1905.

Tanvetyanon T, Bepler G. "Beta-Carotene in Multivitamins and the Possible Risk of Lung Cancer among Smokers Versus Former Smokers: A Meta-Analysis and Evaluation of National Brands." *Cancer* 113 (2008): 150–157.

Multivitamins Keep You Healthy

Avenell A, Campbell MK, Cook JA, et al. "Effect of Multivitamin and Multimineral Supplements on Morbidity from Infections in Older People (MAVIS Trial): Pragmatic, Randomised, Double Blind, Placebo Controlled Trial." *BMJ* 331 (2005): 324–329.

Graat JM, Schouten EG, Kok FJ. "Effect of Daily Vitamin E and Multivitamin-Mineral Supplementation on Acute Respiratory Tract Infections in Elderly Persons: A Randomized Controlled Trial." *Journal of the American Medical Association* 288 (2002): 715–721.

Huang HY, Caballero B, Chang S, et al. "The Efficacy and Safety of Multivitamin and Mineral Supplement Use to Prevent Cancer and Chronic Disease in Adults: A Systematic Review for a National Institutes of Health State-of-the-Science Conference." *Annals of Internal Medicine* 145 (2006): 372–385.

Larsson SC, Akesson A, Bergkvist L, Wolk A. "Multivitamin Use and Breast Cancer Incidence in a Prospective Cohort of Swedish Women." *American Journal of Clinical Nutrition* 91 (2010): 1268–1272.

Lawson KA, Wright ME, Subar A, et al. "Multivitamin Use and Risk of Prostate Cancer in the National Institutes of Health-AARP Diet and Health Study." *Journal of the National Cancer Institute* 99 (2007): 754–764.

Muntwyler J, Hennekens CH, Manson JE, et al. "Vitamin Supplement Use in a Low-Risk Population of US Male Physicians and Subsequent Cardiovascular Mortality." *Archives of Internal Medicine* 162 (2002): 1472–1476.

Neuhouser ML, Wassertheil-Smoller S, Thomson C, et al. "Multivitamin Use and Risk of Cancer and Cardiovascular Disease in the Women's Health Initiative Cohorts." *Archives of Internal Medicine* 169 (2009): 294–304.

Rautiainen S, Akesson A, Levitan EB, et al. "Multivitamin Use and the Risk of Myocardial Infarction: A Population-Based Cohort of Swedish Women." *American Journal of Clinical Nutrition* 92 (2010): 1251–1256.

Stevens VL, McCullough ML, Diver WR, et al. "Use of Multivitamins and Prostate Cancer Mortality in a Large Cohort of US Men." *Cancer Causes & Control* 16 (2005): 643–650.

Stevens VL, McCullough ML, Sun J, Gapstur SM. "Folate and Other One-Carbon Metabolism-Related Nutrients and Risk of Postmenopausal Breast Cancer in the Cancer Prevention Study II Nutrition Cohort." *American Journal of Clinical Nutrition* 91 (2010): 1708–1715.

Stolzenberg-Solomon RZ, Chang SC, Leitzmann MF, et al. "Folate Intake, Alcohol Use, and Postmenopausal Breast Cancer Risk in the Prostate, Lung, Colorectal, and Ovarian Cancer Screening Trial." *American Journal of Clinical Nutrition* 83 (2006): 895–904.

Watkins ML, Erickson JD, Thun MJ, et al. "Multivitamin Use and Mortality in a Large Prospective Study." *American Journal of Epidemiology* 152 (2000): 149–162.

9. SAFE AND SOUND?

Bagged Salad Should Be Washed

"Bagged Salad: How Clean?" *Consumer Reports*, March 2010, p. 15.

Bottled Water Is Safer Than Tap Water

Beverage Marketing Corporation. "Bottled Water Confronts Persist[e]nt Challenges, New Report from Beverage Marketing Corporation Shows." Press release, July 2010.

Lalumandier JA, Ayers LW. "Fluoride and Bacterial Content of Bottled Water Vs. Tap Water." *Archives of Family Medicine* 9 (2000): 246–250.

Naidenko O, Leiba N, Sharp R, Houlihan J. "Bottled Water Quality Investigation: 10 Major Brands, 38 Pollutants." Environmental Working Group, October 15, 2008. www.ewg.org/BottledWater/Bottled-Water-Quality-Investigation/NewsRelease-Response-to-Industry.

Microwaving in Plastic Is Dangerous

Badeka AB, Kontominas MG. "Effect of Microwave Heating on the Migration of Dioctyladipate and Acetyltributylcitrate Plasticizers from Food-Grade PVC and PVDC/PVC Films into Olive Oil and Water." *Zeitschrift für Lebensmittel-Untersuchung und-Forschung* 202 (1996): 313–317.

Halden RU. "Plastics and Health Risks." *Annual Review of Public Health* 31 (2010): 179–194.

Pike-Paris A. "Dissecting an Internet Hoax: Water, Food, Plastics, and Microwaves." *Pediatric Nursing* 31 (2005): 503–507.

Chemicals in French Fries Cause Cancer

Hogervorst JG, Schouten LJ, Konings EJ, et al. "Dietary Acrylamide Intake and the Risk of Renal Cell, Bladder, and Prostate Cancer." *American Journal of Clinical Nutrition* 87 (2008): 1428–1438.

Hogervorst JG, Schouten LJ, Konings EJ, et al. "A Prospective Study of Dietary Acrylamide Intake and the Risk of Endometrial, Ovarian, and Breast Cancer." *Cancer Epidemiology, Biomarkers & Prevention* 16 (2007): 2304–2313.

Larsson SC, Akesson A, Wolk A. "Long-Term Dietary Acrylamide Intake and Risk of Epithelial Ovarian Cancer in a Prospective Cohort of Swedish Women." *Cancer Epidemiology, Biomarkers & Prevention* 18 (2009): 994–997.

Larsson SC, Håkansson N, Akesson A, Wolk A. "Long-Term Dietary Acrylamide Intake and Risk of Endometrial Cancer in a Prospective Cohort of Swedish Women." *International Journal of Cancer* 124 (2009): 1196–1199.

Mulloy KB. "Two Case Reports of Neurological Disease in Coal Mine Preparation Plant Workers." *American Journal of Industrial Medicine* 30 (1996): 56–61.

Olesen PT, Olsen A, Frandsen H, et al. "Acrylamide Exposure and Incidence of Breast Cancer among Postmenopausal Women in the Danish Diet, Cancer and Health Study." *International Journal of Cancer* 122 (2008): 2094–2100.

Pelucchi C, La Vecchia C, Bosetti C, et al. "Exposure to Acrylamide and Human Cancer—A Review and Meta-Analysis of Epidemiologic Studies." *Annals of Oncology* 22 (2011): 1487–1499.

Schouten LJ, Hogervorst JG, Konings EJ, et al. "Dietary Acrylamide Intake and the Risk of Head-Neck and Thyroid Cancers: Results from the Netherlands Cohort Study." *American Journal of Epidemiology* 170 (2009): 873–884.

U.S. Food and Drug Administration. "Survey Data on Acrylamide in Food: Individual Food Products." July 2006. www.fda.gov/food/foodsafety/foodcontam inantsadulteration/chemicalcontaminants/acrylamide/ucm053549.htm.

Wilson KM, Mucci LA, Cho E, et al. Dietary Acrylamide Intake and Risk of Premenopausal Breast Cancer." *American Journal of Epidemiology* 169 (2009): 954–961.

Genetically Modified Foods Are Harmful

Centers for Disease Control and Prevention. "Investigation of Human Health Effects Associated with Potential Exposure to Genetically Modified Corn: A Report to the U.S. Food and Drug Administration from the Centers for Disease Control and Prevention." June 11, 2001. www.cdc.gov/nceh/ehhe/cry9creport/pdfs/cry9creport.pdf.

Domingo JL. "Toxicity Studies of Genetically Modified Plants: A Review of the Published Literature." *Critical Reviews in Food Science and Nutrition* 47 (2007): 721–733.

Ewen SW, Pusztai A. "Effect of Diets Containing Genetically Modified Potatoes Expressing *Galanthus nivalis* Lectin on Rat Small Intestine." *Lancet* 354 (1999): 1353–1354.

Key S, Ma JK, Drake PM. "Genetically Modified Plants and Human Health." *Journal of the Royal Society of Medicine* 101 (2008): 290–298.

Nordlee JA, Taylor SL, Townsend JA, et al. "Identification of a Brazil-Nut Allergen in Transgenic Soybeans." *New England Journal of Medicine* 334 (1996): 688–692.

Royal Society. "Review of Data on Possible Toxicity of GM Potatoes." June 1999. http://royalsociety.org/Review-of-data-on-possible-toxicity-of-GM-potatoes.

Thomson Reuters. *National Survey of Healthcare Consumers: Genetically Engineered Food.* October 2010. www.factsforhealthcare.com/pressroom/NPR_report _GeneticEngineeredFood.pdf.

Irradiated Food Is Unsafe

O'Bryan CA, Crandall PG, Ricke SC, Olson DG. "Impact of Irradiation on the Safety and Quality of Poultry and Meat Products: A Review." *Critical Reviews in Food Science and Nutrition* 48 (2008): 442–457.

Osterholm MT, Norgan AP. "The Role of Irradiation in Food Safety." *New England Journal of Medicine* 350 (2004): 1898–1901.

Raul F, Gosse F, Delincee H, et al. "Food-Borne Radiolytic Compounds (2-Alkylcy-clobutanones) May Promote Experimental Colon Carcinogenesis." *Nutrition and Cancer* 44 (2002): 189–191.

Tauxe RV. "Food Safety and Irradiation: Protecting the Public from Foodborne Infections." *Emerging Infectious Diseases* 7 [Suppl 3] (2001): 516–521.

10. DIET DOCTRINES

Vegetarian Diets Are More Healthful Than Other Diets

Appleby P, Roddam A, Allen N, Key T. "Comparative Fracture Risk in Vegetarians and Nonvegetarians in EPIC-Oxford." *European Journal of Clinical Nutrition* 61 (2007): 1400–1406.

Craig WJ. "Health Effects of Vegan Diets." *American Journal of Clinical Nutrition* 89 (2009): 1627S–1633S.

Fraser GE. "Vegetarian Diets: What Do We Know of Their Effects on Common Chronic Diseases?" *American Journal of Clinical Nutrition* 89 (2009): 1607S–1612S.

Key TJ, Appleby PN, Rosell MS. "Health Effects of Vegetarian and Vegan Diets." *Proceedings of the Nutrition Society* 65 (2006): 35–41.

Key TJ, Appleby PN, Spencer EA, et al. "Cancer Incidence in British Vegetarians." *British Journal of Cancer* 101 (2009): 192–197.

A Mediterranean Diet Is Good for You

Baron KG, Reid KJ, Kern AS, Zee PC. "Role of Sleep Timing in Caloric Intake and BMI." *Obesity* (Silver Spring) 19 (2011): 1374–1381.

de Lorgeril M, Salen P, Martin JL, et al. "Mediterranean Diet, Traditional Risk Factors, and the Rate of Cardiovascular Complications after Myocardial Infarction: Final Report of the Lyon Diet Heart Study." *Circulation* 99 (1999): 779–785.

Esposito K, Maiorino MI, Ceriello A, Giugliano D. "Prevention and Control of Type 2 Diabetes by Mediterranean Diet: A Systematic Review." *Diabetes Research and Clinical Practice* 89 (2010): 97–102.

Esposito K, Marfella R, Ciotola M, et al. "Effect of a Mediterranean-Style Diet on Endothelial Dysfunction and Markers of Vascular Inflammation in the Metabolic Syndrome: A Randomized Trial." *Journal of the American Medical Association* 292 (2004): 1440–1446.

Kant AK, Schatzkin A, Ballard-Barbash R. "Evening Eating and Subsequent Long-Term Weight Change in a National Cohort." *International Journal of Obesity and Related Metabolic Disorders* 21 (1997): 407–412.

Kastorini CM, Milionis HJ, Goudevenos JA, Panagiotakos DB. "Mediterranean Diet and Coronary Heart Disease: Is Obesity a Link? A Systematic Review." *Nutrition, Metabolism & Cardiovascular Diseases* 20 (2010): 536–551.

Serra-Majem L, Roman B, Estruch R. "Scientific Evidence of Interventions Using the Mediterranean Diet: A Systematic Review." *Nutrition Reviews* 64 [Part 2] (2006): S27–S47.

Shai I, Schwarzfuchs D, Henkin Y, et al. "Weight Loss with a Low-Carbohydrate, Mediterranean, or Low-Fat Diet." *New England Journal of Medicine* 359 (2008): 229–241.

Sofi F, Abbate R, Gensini GF, Casini A. "Accruing Evidence about Benefits of Adherence to the Mediterranean Diet on Health: An Updated Systematic Review and Meta-Analysis." *American Journal of Clinical Nutrition* 92 (2010): 1189–1196.

Tambalis KD, Panagiotakos DB, Kavouras SA, et al. "Eleven-Year Prevalence Trends of Obesity in Greek Children: First Evidence That Prevalence of Obesity Is Leveling Off." *Obesity* (Silver Spring) 18 (2010): 161–166.

Trichopoulou A, Bamia C, Trichopoulos D. "Anatomy of Health Effects of Mediterranean Diet: Greek EPIC Prospective Cohort Study." *BMJ* 23 (2009): b2337.

Detox Diets Make You Healthier

Boseley S. "'Make-Believe and Outright Quackery'—Expert's Verdict on Prince's Detox Potion." *Guardian*, March 11, 2009.

Duchy Herbals Detox Tincture, www.duchyoriginals.com/detox_tincture.php.

A Caveman Diet Is Ideal

Frassetto LA, Schloetter M, Mietus-Synder M, et al. "Metabolic and Physiologic Improvements from Consuming a Paleolithic, Hunter-Gatherer Type Diet." *European Journal of Clinical Nutrition* 63 (2009): 947–955.

Jönsson T, Granfeldt Y, Ahrén B, et al. "Beneficial Effects of a Paleolithic Diet on Cardiovascular Risk Factors in Type 2 Diabetes: A Randomized Cross-Over Pilot Study." *Cardiovascular Diabetology* 8 (2009): 35.

Lindeberg S, Jönsson T, Granfeldt Y, et al. "A Palaeolithic Diet Improves Glucose Tolerance More Than a Mediterranean-Like Diet in Individuals with Ischaemic Heart Disease." *Diabetologia* 50 (2007): 1795–1807.

Lindeberg S, Lundh B. "Apparent Absence of Stroke and Ischaemic Heart Disease in a Traditional Melanesian Island: A Clinical Study in Kitava." *Journal of Internal Medicine* 233 (1993): 269–275.

Osterdahl M, Kocturk T, Koochek A, Wändell PE. "Effects of a Short-Term Intervention with a Paleolithic Diet in Healthy Volunteers." *European Journal of Clinical Nutrition* 62 (2008): 682–685.

Diets High in Watery Foods Help You Lose Weight

Bes-Rastrollo M, van Dam RM, Martinez-Gonzalez MA, et al. "Prospective Study of Dietary Energy Density and Weight Gain in Women." *American Journal of Clinical Nutrition* 88 (2008): 769–777.

Blatt AD, Roe LS, Rolls BJ. "Hidden Vegetables: An Effective Strategy to Reduce Energy Intake and Increase Vegetable Intake in Adults." *American Journal of Clinical Nutrition* 93 (2011): 756–763.

Ello-Martin JA, Roe LS, Ledikwe JH, et al. "Dietary Energy Density in the Treatment of Obesity: A Year-Long Trial Comparing 2 Weight-Loss Diets." *American Journal of Clinical Nutrition* 85 (2007): 1465–1477.

Ledikwe JH, Rolls BJ, Smiciklas-Wright H, et al. "Reductions in Dietary Energy Density Are Associated with Weight Loss in Overweight and Obese Participants in the PREMIER Trial." *American Journal of Clinical Nutrition* 85 (2007): 1212–1221.

Rolls BJ. "The Relationship between Dietary Energy Density and Energy Intake." *Physiology & Behavior* 97 (2009): 609–615.

Rolls B. *The Volumetrics Eating Plan: Techniques and Recipes for Feeling Full on Fewer Calories.* New York: HarperCollins, 2004.

Rolls BJ, Roe LS, Beach AM, Kris-Etherton PM. "Provision of Foods Differing in Energy Density Affects Long-Term Weight Loss." *Obesity Research* 13 (2005): 1052–1060.

Seinfield J. *Deceptively Delicious: Simple Secrets to Get Your Kids Eating Good Food.* New York: HarperCollins, 2007.

Very Low Calorie Diets Extend Your Life

Colman RJ, Anderson RM, Johnson SC, et al. "Caloric Restriction Delays Disease Onset and Mortality in Rhesus Monkeys." *Science* 325 (2009): 201–204.

Dirks AJ, Leeuwenburgh C. "Caloric Restriction in Humans: Potential Pitfalls and Health Concerns." *Mechanisms of Ageing and Development* 127 (2006): 1–7.

Flegal KM, Graubard BI, Williamson DF, Gail MH. "Cause-Specific Excess Deaths Associated with Underweight, Overweight, and Obesity." *Journal of the American Medical Association* 298 (2007): 2028–2037.

Fontana L, Klein S. "Aging, Adiposity, and Calorie Restriction." *Journal of the American Medical Association* 297 (2007): 986–994.

Fontana L, Meyer TE, Klein S, Holloszy JO. "Long-Term Calorie Restriction Is Highly Effective in Reducing the Risk for Atherosclerosis in Humans." *Proceedings of the National Academy of Sciences of the United States of America* 101 (2004): 6659–6663.

Heilbronn LK, de Jonge L, Frisard MI, et al. "Effect of 6-Month Calorie Restriction on Biomarkers of Longevity, Metabolic Adaptation, and Oxidative Stress in Overweight Individuals: A Randomized Controlled Trial." *Journal of the American Medical Association* 295 (2006): 1539–1548.

Varady KA, Hellerstein MK. "Alternate-Day Fasting and Chronic Disease Prevention: A Review of Human and Animal Trials." *American Journal of Clinical Nutrition* 86 (2007): 7–13.

Index

Page numbers in *italics* indicate figures.

About the Author

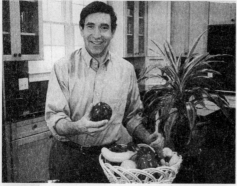

Mria Dangerfield

Robert J. Davis, PhD, is an award-winning health journalist whose work has appeared on CNN, PBS, and WebMD, and in the *Wall Street Journal*. He is founder and editor in chief of Everwell.com and the author of *The Healthy Skeptic*. He also teaches at Emory University's Rollins School of Public Health. A graduate of Princeton University, he holds a master's degree in public health from Emory and a PhD in health policy from Brandeis University, where he was a Pew Foundation Fellow.